THE STRENGTH TRAINING PROTOCOL

Gain Strength And Muscle Growth in 10 Days

Logan Legend

Table of Contents

Introduction..7
Chapter 1: How to Choose the Right Number of Repetitions................8
Chapter 2: How to Breathe During Exercises......................................11
Chapter 3: Machines or Free Weights?...13
Chapter 4: Putting it all together. How to program a training cycle......16

PART 2..20
Chapter 1: Setting Yourself Up For Success.....................................21
Chapter 2: Types of Bodyweight Workouts.......................................26
Chapter 3: Planning a Workout Routine That Works For You.............32
Chapter 4: How to Make the Most Out of Your Bodyweight Workouts......37

PART 3..39
Chapter One: Muscle Mass..40
   How Muscle is Built..41
Chapter Two: The Upper Body...42
   1. The Classic Push-Up..42
   2. Chair-Dips..43
   3. Diamond Push-Ups...43
Chapter Three: The Core...45
   4. Plank...46
   5. Reverse Crunch...47
   6. Mountain Climber..48
Chapter Four: The Lower Body..49
   7. The Lunge..50
   8. Squat...51
   9. The Bridge...51
Chapter Five: Putting it all Together..53
Chapter Six: On Your Diet...56

PART 4..58
PART 4.1: What Is Fasting and Why You Should Do it..............59
Chapter 1: What Is Fasting?...60
Introduction to Fasting..60
Latest Research and Studies about Fasting.........................60
Biological Effects of Fasting...61
Treating Fasting as a Lifestyle Choice...............................62
Summary..63
Chapter 2: Obesity and the Standard American Diet................64
The Obesity Epidemic...64
Why Are We So Fat?...65
The Problem with Calories...66
The American Diet...67
Summary..68
Chapter 3: Benefits of Fasting..69
Summary..80
Chapter 4: Myths and Dangers of Fasting............................82
Long-Held Myths and Misconceptions about Fasting............82
Busting Myths Associated with Fasting.............................82
Dangers of Fasting...83
Summary..84
Chapter 5: Safety, Side Effects, and Warning.......................86
The Safest and Enlightened Way of Fasting.......................86
Side Effects of Fasting..86
Types of People That Should Not Fast..............................88
Summary..89

PART 4.2: Types of Fasting and How to Fast......................90
Chapter 6: Intermittent Fasting..91

- What Is Intermittent Fasting?..........91
- How to Practice Intermittent Fasting..........91
- Pros and Cons of Intermittent Fasting..........92
- Finding Your Ideal Intermittent Fasting Plan..........93
- Step-By-Step Process of Fasting For a Week..........94
- Summary..........96

Chapter 7: Longer Periods of Fasting..........97
- What is Fasting for Longer Periods?..........97
- How to Fast for Longer Periods..........97
- Pros and Cons of Fasting for Longer Periods..........98
- Step-By-Step Process of Fasting for Longer Periods..........99
- Preparation..........99

Chapter 8: Extended Fasting..........101
- How to Fast for Extended Periods..........101
- Pros and Cons of Fasting for Extended Periods..........101
- Step-By-Step Process of Fasting for Extended Periods..........102

Chapter 9: The Eating Window..........104
- What is the Eating Window?..........104
- What to Eat..........105
- Developing Discipline..........106
- Summary..........106

PART 4.3: Targeted Fasting for Your Body Type..........108
Chapter 10: Fasting For Weight Loss..........109
- Why You'll Lose Weight through Fasting..........109
- Step-By-Step Process of Losing Weight through Fasting..........110
- Summary..........112

Chapter 11: Fasting for Type 2 Diabetes..........113
- What is Type 2 Diabetes?..........113

- The Role of Insulin in the Body..114
- How Diabetes Affects both Production and Usage of Insulin...115
- How Blood Sugar Responds To Fasting..................................116
- Developing Your Fasting Regimen..116
- Things to Incorporate to Make Fasting Safe for Diabetics..........117
- Role of Supplements...118
- Types of Supplements that Stabilize Electrolytes......................119
- How to Keep Insulin Levels Low...120
- What Causes Insulin Resistance?..121
- How Insulin Resistance Affects the Body..................................122
- The Role of Amylin..123
- How Amylin Deficiency Affects Your Body.............................123
- The Insulin Resistance Diet...124
- The Best Food for Diabetics..125
- Summary...126

Chapter 12: Fasting For Heart Health...127
- How Fasting Improves Your Heart's Health...............................127
- Summary...128

Chapter 13: The General Results of Fasting..................................129
- Positive Effects of Fasting...129
- Negative Effects of Fasting...130
- Summary...130

PART 4.4 Important Factors that Improve the Quality of Fasting....132

Chapter 14: Nutrition...133
- What Constitutes Good Nutrition?..133
- Why Good Nutrition Is Important...134
- The Advantages of a High-Fat Diet..135
- Role of Ketone Bodies...136

- Benefits of the Ketogenic Diet..137
- The Importance of a Well-Balanced Diet..................................138
- Summary...139

Chapter 15: Exercise..140
- Pros of Exercising While Fasting..140
- Best Exercises to Do..141
- Summary...142

Chapter 16: Having a Partner to Keep You in Check......................143
- Role of a Partner..143
- Traits to Look for in a Partner...143
- Should You Join A Support Group?..144
- Summary...145

Chapter 17: Motivation..147
- How to Stay Motivated Throughout Your Fast.......................147
- How to Make Fasting Your Lifestyle...148
- Summary...149

Chapter 18: Foods for the Fast...150
- How Food Controls the Rate of the Success of Fasting.............150
- The Worst Foods to Take During Fasting................................151
- The Best Foods to Take During Fasting...................................152
- Summary...153

Conclusion...154

Introduction

The world of strength training is growing increasingly chaotic, and downloading this book is the first step you can take towards getting a little bit more clarity about it. The first step is also always the easiest, which is why the information you find in the following chapters is so important to take to heart as they are not concepts that can be put into action immediately. If you file them away for when they are really needed in the gym, however, then when the time comes to use them, you will be glad you did learn them. What I have discovered after years of strength training, in fact, is that most people think that there is no theoretical aspect behind the exercises they are performing. Instead, knowing it is extremely important to acquiring a better form.

To that end, the following chapters will discuss the primary preparedness principals that you will need to consider if you ever hope to be ready to build up your strength over a period of time. Only by having the right knowledge will you be able to lay out a clear plan to get bigger, leaner and stronger.

In this book, you will learn everything you need to know about strength training and how to take your gains to the next level. The same principles have helped hundreds of other people and me to get the body they desired.

There are plenty of books on this subject on the market. Thanks again for choosing this one! Every effort was made to ensure it is full of as much useful information as possible. Please enjoy!

Chapter 1: How to Choose the Right Number of Repetitions

"How do I choose the number of repetitions and series?"

This is one of the main doubts that assail the neophytes of the gym. I still remember the day I asked my gym instructor about it many years ago. In fact, the first questions that a beginner poses to the instructor in front of a weight machine are typically these: "How many consecutive lifts (or movements) do I have to do with this machines? And for how many times?"

The most precise ones even dare to ask how much time they have to recover from one set to the next one, and so you think you have clarified everything you need to know about a training session at a given weight machine.

The load (i.e., the kg lifted or moved) is generally fixed according to the presumed abilities of the aspiring visitor of the weight room, often without any relation to the first two parameters of repetitions and sets.

There is not a unique answer to these questions since it all depends on the goal. For example, when I first started my training journey, I wanted to get bigger, not stronger. During that period I did a lot of hypertrophy-oriented workouts which worked quite well. When I switched to a more strength-oriented approach, I had to completely rearrange my schedule all over again.

Since the weight training that interests us is not aimed at the practice of bodybuilding—but is framed in the health of those who want to integrate aerobic activities with exercises for the general improvement of strength, elasticity, and flexibility—before defining the number of repetitions and sets, it is necessary to establish the objective to be achieved or what aspect do you want to train for between the following:

- **The resistant force**: the force that the muscle must apply to overcome the fatigue resulting from a prolonged effort.

- **The maximal force**: the maximum force that the muscle can develop with a lifting test (or a limited number of tests). It is also often referred to as a maximal load if referring to a specific exercise in the gym.

- **The fast force:** the maximum force that the muscle can develop to counteract a load in a limited period of time. Referring to time, therefore, more than force we should speak of power which is the ability to develop a force in the unity of time.

- **Muscle hypertrophy**: no reference is made to the type of force that the muscle has to generate, but to its effect on the athlete's body—that is, to maximize the increase in muscle volume. The muscular volume is connected to the developed force, because the greater the cross section of the muscle, the greater the muscle fibers available to make the effort. However, the equation *muscle hypertrophy = greater muscle strength* is not always true because, in addition to having available muscle fibers, the human body must also know how to recruit, and this is influenced by other factors such as the efficiency of the cardio-respiratory system, the ability coordination, etc. This should make those who seek to maximize muscle hypertrophy think only of achieving the highest possible performance.

In a healthy view of strength training, you can leave out the last point because the search for muscle hypertrophy, typical of bodybuilders, is far from our goals. Therefore, we can identify three types of training, each of which corresponds to a type of strength that you want to train and, consequently, to a pattern of repetitions-number of sets-interval between the different series.

Remember that to define a training plan, the following variables must be defined for each exercise (i.e., for each machine in the gym or exercise with weights):

- Repetition: it is the single gesture of weightlifting or athletic gesture that stresses the muscle or a district of the muscles. Generally, in the gym at each repetition, the muscle or muscles lift or move a weight (load).

- Sets: the consecutive number of repetitions. The set can be slow or fast, or the exercise is done slowly, calmly, or quickly, imposing to adhere to a higher rhythm.

- Recovery: the time between one series and the next.

So, you might find a typical 3-row workout of 12 sets of 25 kg with a three-minute recovery. This is a very standard way to get started and the first style of training that I followed when started out.

Chapter 2: How to Breathe During Exercises

One thing that is often overlooked by many gym enthusiasts is how to perform proper breathing during weight exercises. It is a problem that, sooner or later, most of those who attend gyms propose to their instructor.

Breathing, as we know, is an activity that we do involuntarily, but it is also possible to control it trying to adapt the movement of the muscles (or part of the muscles) involved, such as the diaphragm, the ribcage, the shoulders, abdominals to the rhythm that we want to follow.

Consciously, one can control the inhalation phase and the exhalation phase in their overall duration or even suspend breathing by entering apnoea.

A lot of sports and disciplines (yoga, pilates, etc.), give a lot of importance to breathing, while other oriental disciplines even give it a spiritual value.

Even in the exercises that are performed in the gym, including those with weights, breathing has a considerable importance. Unfortunately, there are not many who have clear ideas about it.

Instructors usually advise to:

- **inhale** in the discharge phase of the action, usually when the weight is being returned to its initial position;
- **exhale** in the loading phase of the exercise or when there is more effort required.

This usually works well, even if the beginner will at first see this as another constraint which will only confuse him. In reality, it requires a good amount of concentration to force yourself to control breathing in this way and therefore forces the athlete to give complete attention to what he is doing. A lot of times, people look around in the gym while doing an exercise, or—worse—talking to someone. This is something that I have never understood: to me, strength training is a way to become the best version of myself, both physically and mentally, and I do not have time to waste. Focusing on breathing is a good way to think exclusively about the exercise you are performing.

The following is a good general rule to follow:

The most important thing to do is not to hold your breath during the loading phase.

Holding your breath in the loading phase is a big mistake, as it is instinctive to hold your breath during the maximum effort required. Instead, the opposite must be done because this practice can also lead to serious consequences, especially if the effort involves muscles of the upper body.

Holding the breath deliberately blocks the glottis, which then leads to a compression of the veins due to an increase in pressure inside the ribcage. As a result of this compression, the veins can also partially occlude (as if they were strangled by one hand) and this considerably slows the return of venous blood to the heart. As a consequence, the arterial pressure rises, reaching even impressive values such as 300 mmHg (usually 120 mmHg at rest). Moreover, as a consequence of the reduced blood supply to the heart, the outgoing blood also slows down and reduces, which decreases the blood and oxygen supply to the peripheral organs. Less blood and oxygen to the brain could result in dizziness, blurred vision, etc. until you eventually faint. These are side effects well-known by opera singers who practice hyperventilation exercises that, in some parts, are performed in apnoea.

Chapter 3: Machines or Free Weights?

The question is interesting, and the purpose of this chapter is to precisely evaluate the advantages and disadvantages of two possible training solutions for muscle strengthening: the use of gym machines or exercise with the aid of free weights.

From a health point of view, it is clear that the question of the title seems reasonable because, unlike in a bodybuilder, muscle strengthening is seen only as a preparatory to a sport or as a general improvement of the body, and therefore it is not said that the use of gym machines is actually the only possible solution for those who want to make a good upgrade without wanting to reach professional levels of a bodybuilding lover. Before analyzing the two solutions in detail, briefly remember that a muscle can perform an effort in two ways of contraction: eccentric or concentric.

In the first case, the muscle develops the force necessary for the exercise when it is stretching, in the second case when it is being shortened.

Weights and machines are not always equivalent in stimulating a muscle in an eccentric and concentric way. For the purpose of training, eccentric work is the most difficult—to the point that it can also induce pain and muscle damage. It is therefore important that, by deciding which exercises to perform (with the machines or with the weights), it is clear (otherwise you can ask the instructor like I did at the beginning of my journey in the gym) which exercises stimulate the muscles more eccentrically, to introduce them gradually into the plan of training avoiding injuries.

Weight Machines

In the gym, there are usually many weight machines. Generally, except for the multi-function stations, each of them trains a specific muscular district or even a single type of muscle. The effort put in place by the muscles during the execution of the exercise must counteract two physical forces: the weight force and the force due to the friction of the weight that it moves (often along ropes or pulleys).

As a general rule of the mechanics involved in the use of weights, during the eccentric contraction, the friction force is subtracted from that of the weight, while during the concentric contraction this force is added.

Free Weights

They are called free-weight exercises because usually the weights are not tied to ropes or pulleys of the machines, but simply gripped or tied to the body (for example with anklets) and carried out only with the aid of weights such as dumbbells and barbells, which are often seen on sale in supermarkets. Surely, compared to a workout with machines, the one with free weights is easier to put in place. Often, it is not even necessary to attend a gym; a small home space equipped with a mat, a bench (if required by the exercises), a mirror (optional, to control the movements) and, of course, the weights is sufficient enough.

Now let's analyze the advantages and disadvantages of the two solutions, taking into consideration some objective parameters that can assume different importance depending on the individual's objectives, the physical state of departure (sedentary, beginner or advanced athlete), and the expectations placed in a training of this type.

- Economic aspect: free weight training is certainly cheaper, because, as mentioned, in most cases it is not necessary to get a gym subscription. It can be a good compromise solution to go to the gym for the time necessary to practice the exercises under the guidance of an experienced instructor, and then, once you are sure to perform the correct movements, buy weights and equip yourself with a training-space inside your home. This is what I did, and I would never go back.

- Versatility: free weights are suitable for multiple exercises and different muscle groups. Think about how many exercises you can do with simple weights to train biceps, triceps, pectorals, etc. In the case of training with weight machines, each machine usually allows a few exercises (if not only one) and this is the practical limit of such a training: you need to choose a gym where there is a sufficient number of machines for the exercises you want to do and where waiting times are not too long. Otherwise, the queues to the machines make the overall workout boring and ineffective.

- Eccentric and concentric training: weight machines usually lesser stress the eccentric work of the muscle (because of the opposing frictional force) unlike the movement of the body which, in returning to the starting position of the exercise, often performs eccentric work of considerable intensity. Moreover, in the exercises with weights, many antagonistic muscles are trained many times, and in general, they also train the balance and proprioceptive, improving body coordination.

- Safety and complexity: from the previous point, we can see that weight machines train specific muscle areas, and it is easier to isolate the muscle or muscle district involved. It is also easier to perform the exercise correctly because the movements are constrained by the machines and are easier to learn. With free weights, it is easier to make mistakes, and generally more antagonistic muscles and the spine are stimulated. In addition, with the weights, it is easier to maintain a constant execution speed. For all these reasons, it is generally said that the exercises with the machines are at a lower risk of injury than those with free weights.

Chapter 4: Putting it all together. How to program a training cycle

Now we come to the crucial point: how do I craft a strength training program? The question is very complex. Each strategy will be based on the condition of the subject, so, logically, when we see a disproportionate lack of strength for a muscle group, it will be logical to intervene in this sense. Let's go step by step. The literature on the subject highlights how, for the purposes of muscular hypertrophy and gains in strength, setting a periodized program is the best solution. Before diving deeper into the topic, it is important to note something. You cannot generalize, there is no way to use a unique approach or way of training a particular component. There are countless cases, solutions. So what can be done is to report different models based on different contexts to give not a guide but a concept—something infinitely more precious (and expendable).

Strategy 1. "Basic" Approach. A first approach that we can use is to set up a multifrequency workout by adopting a daily wavy periodization. So we will have two weekly sessions for each muscle district. In the first session we can train the muscle according to a traditional bodybuilding scheme, then longer TUT, intensity techniques, a range of 8-12 repetitions, eccentric, forced, etc. In the second session, we can train ourselves by adopting a progression of strength. So for example, we will train the chest on a flat bench using possibly another complementary exercise (like crosses, chest fly, etc.). A similar approach is at the base of the PHAT (Power Hypertrophy Adaptive Training) method proposed by Norton. Unlike this, however, I find it more sensible to use—in training dedicated to strength—real progressions on exercises without being limited to a 5 × 5 standard type of training.

Strategy 2. Deficient Muscles Approach. Similar to the previous one, the only difference is that a workout in this sense will be done on the deficient muscles while the more developed muscles will be trained in monofrequency. The increase in weekly volume and stimulus variation will bring an advantage in terms of growth (strength and hypertrophy) that will allow you to "catch up" with respect to the rest of the muscles. This approach can be used on deficient muscles both from a hypertrophy point of view and from a force point of view (i.e., the weakest muscles). This last aspect is particularly important as it can be a valid strategy to intervene where a muscle is placed limiting within the synergy of a gesture. The discourse can also be done from the opposite point of view —that is, to hold the strongest or most developed muscle groups to a multifrequency and to mono-frequency to recover asymmetries (aesthetic or functional).

Strategy 3. The transient phase of reduced volume. Another way to insert a strength training within a bodybuilding program is to provide a period with a high load intensity and a reduced volume. In this case, we always speak of wavy periodization. However, the variations will not be done on a daily basis, but weekly. So, for instance, we will put 2-3 up to 6 weeks of strength training with a reduced volume—less dense workouts but with the intensity of high-load and then return, progressively or not, to traditional bodybuilding sessions, or even to a wavy periodization protocol on a daily basis as described above. Basically, it is a matter of setting a transitional phase aimed at two purposes: Varying the stimulus (Ri) and finding the feeling with the motor scheme.

Strategy 4. Periodization within the session. This is also an interesting approach. It is a matter of inserting, within the session, an exercise on which to set up a forced schedule. In this sense, we could then insert the flat bench into a chest session as a first or second exercise. We will choose a program to improve on strength (since we are already able to exercise the right mastery over the exercise) and set the rest of the session as a traditional bodybuilding session. Obviously, the total volume will decrease as part of the session is occupied by dense work—not very voluminous but very intense. I find that such a setting fits well with the daily wavy periodization (strategy 1). Basically, by training a multi-frequency muscle, we will set the strength session using an exercise with its progression and the rest of the session in the traditional bodybuilding style. The diversification of work with respect to the second weekly session will be in the TUT (for example) which, in the latter, will be exasperated (e.g.,

+50'), while in the session of "strength" it will not be too high (e.g., 30').

Split and choice of exercises

A further aspect on which we must dwell is that relative to the decision, within the session, the target muscle groups and the exercises to be used. One of the characteristics of strength programs is that, in most cases, the various muscle groups are subdivided to work only a few each session. This is logical because the work that is required is always of the same type (anaerobic). Okay, as we have seen, it can work on different adaptive components, but in any case, it is always part of the big family of "boosting" work, the same that, in other sports, is alternated with "technical" work. The question that arises is the following: Should we first set the split and then, based on this, choose the type of exercises in which to work the strength or vice versa? Being a powerlifter myself, I would answer "the second," but from a Bodybuilder perspective I would answer "the first." Since this chapter is about strength training, I would say start from this context and, in particular, from the cases mentioned above. Where we want to set a wavy periodization, for all groups or only for some (strategies 1-2-4), then yes, we will have to start from the split. Based on this we will choose the best exercise on which to progress for the strength. So for example, in a push-day, we will choose the Bench Press for the chest, for a pull-day a Bent Over Row, and for a leg-day a Squat.

Let's do an example: Subject 1, Powerlifter, good management of high loads on the various motor schemes. Deficient groups: Arms, Back. Strong groups: Chest, Quadriceps

Split

Day 1 Push Day

Day 2 Pull Day

Day 3 Leg Day

Day 4 Rest

Day 5 Arms

Day 6 Back

Day 7 Glutes

Logically, we will then insert a progression on the Bent-Over Row on day 2 and work the Back with a traditional strength session on day 6. To evaluate a progression on the ground clearance that would be close to a leg workout (even putting it on day 6), we will have the hamstrings on day 7. But training strength, as we have seen, is not just a matter of periodizing and varying the stimulus, but also a question of functionality to the motor schemes to be performed during the sessions.

So let's take another example. Subject 2: Powerlifter, poor activation of the chest on the bench press, poor feeling on the deadlift. Excellent management of the Squat. Deficient groups: Chest-Back-Arms. The goal, in this case, will be to improve the feeling with easier exercises so we will set the split based on the same.

Split

Day 1 Chest and Shoulders

Day 2 Deadlift day

Day 3 Rest

Day 4 Quadriceps and Arms

Day 5 Rest

Day 6 Chest and Back

Day 7 Arms

Finally, in case we go set up a Strength program as a transitory phase (strategy 3), it will be logical to start from the exercises and, based on these, reason on the split.

PART 2

Chapter 1: Setting Yourself Up For Success

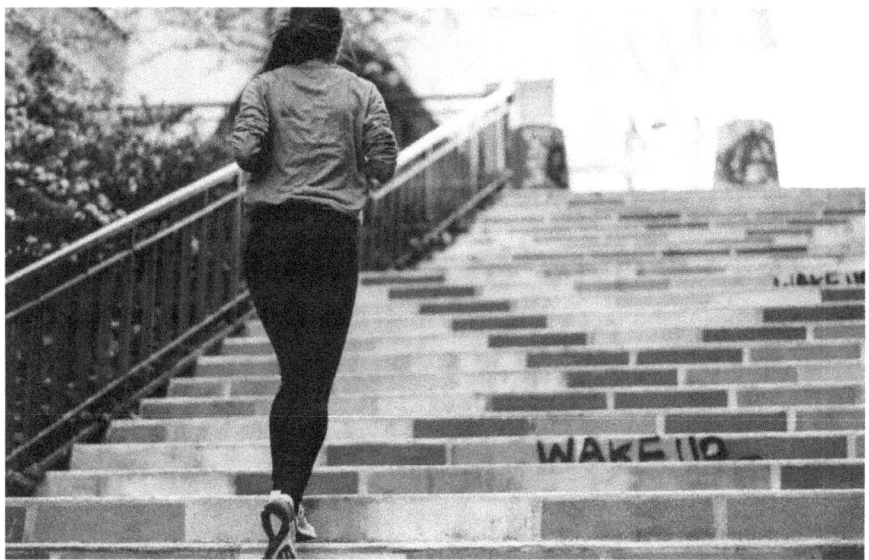

Photo byEvonUnsplash

How Your Diet Affects Your Results

Exercise and diet are equally important factors to building muscle and losing fat. It is generally touted that diet may even play a larger role in the outcome of your fitness. If you are working out hard and not seeing results, make sure that the things you are eating are unprocessed and have high nutrient values—more specifically, work with a nutritionist to find the macronutrient intake levels that are right for the goal you are trying to reach.

Warm Up Before Working Out

To avoid injury, we should take some time before starting our workout to warm up all of our muscle groups. It is generally accepted that warming up before a workout will lead to better performance results and decrease the chance of injuring yourself. Don't forget to stretch after you're done, too! Warming up and cooling down should take no less than 5 minutes, but no more than 15-20 minutes. We don't want all your time spent prepping for your workout or stretching afterward, but they are important components that ensure your body's continued functionality.

Example Warm Up Workouts:

Complete these exercises for 5-10 minutes

1. Jog, row, or ride a bike at a slow-medium pace
2. Jump rope
3. High knees or butt kicks
4. Walk-out planks
5. Jumping jacks

Important Areas to Stretch:

Areas are followed by examples

1. Arms: arm circles
2. Legs: walking lunges
3. Glutes: glute bridge
4. Calves: wall lean
5. Back: leg pull

When warming up, we want our heart rate to increase, so make sure that while you are completing these exercises, you are adequately exerting yourself. We want our body to be ready for the more intense activity we are about to take part in. An increase in blood flow, an increase in body temperature, and an increase in breathing rate all build slowly through warming up in preparation. If you need to ask yourself if you are working out vigorously enough, a good test to check is to see if you would be able to keep a conversation going with your friend. If you are working out hard enough, you really shouldn't be able to keep a conversation going.

Who These Workouts Are Best-Suited For

Bodyweight Workouts are best-suited for those who cannot afford a gym membership, don't enjoy the gym atmosphere, or for those who feel like they are too large to jump right into fast-paced routines. Memberships can be expensive depending on where you go, and we don't all have enough money to afford one at certain points in our lives. Many people—women, in particular—feel uncomfortable at the gym or are intimidated by the size of the facility and the variety of equipment. Bodyweight Workouts can be modified for someone of any shape and size and can be completed in the privacy of your own home if you are self-conscious by working out in public.

Benefits of Bodyweight Workouts

These workouts allow you to build muscle, gain strength, and increase your stamina by using nothing other than your body. Able to be completed anywhere and with no equipment, Bodyweight Workouts are fast and effective. The Huffington Post contributor Dave Smith lists the numerous benefits of Bodyweight Workouts:

1. <u>They are efficient</u>: "Research suggests high-output, bodyweight-based exercises such as plyometrics yield awesome fitness gains in very short workout durations. Since there's no equipment involved, bodyweight workouts make it easy to transition quickly from one exercise to the next. Shorter rest times mean it's easy to boost heart rate and burn some serious calories quickly."

2. <u>There's something for everyone</u>: "Bodyweight exercises are a great choice because they're easily modified to challenge any fitness level. Adding extra repetitions, performing the exercises faster or super-slow, and perfecting form are a few ways to make even the simplest exercise more challenging. And progress is easy to measure since bodyweight exercises offer endless ways to do a little more in each workout."

3. <u>They can improve core strength</u>: "The 'core' is not just the abs. At least 29 muscles make up our core. Many bodyweight movements can be used to engage all of them. These will improve core strength, resulting in better posture and improved athletic performance."

4. <u>Workouts are convenient</u>: "Ask someone why they don't exercise. Chances are they'll answer they have 'no time' or that it's an 'inconvenience.' These common obstacles are eliminated by bodyweight exercises because they allow anyone to squeeze in workouts any time, anywhere. It can be a stress reliever for those who work at home, or it can be a great hotel room workout for people on the road. With bodyweight workouts, 'no time' becomes no excuse."

5. <u>Workouts can be fun and easily mixed up for variety:</u> "It can be easy to get stuck in a workout rut of bench presses, lat pull-downs, and biceps curls. That's why bodyweight training can be so refreshing: There are countless exercise variations that can spice up any workout routine. Working with a variety of exercises not only relieves potential workout boredom, but it can also help break through exercise plateaus to spark further fitness progress."

6. <u>They can provide quick results</u>: "Bodyweight exercises get results partly because they often involve compound movements. Compound exercises such as push-ups, lunges, and chin-ups have been shown to be extremely effective for strength gains and performance improvements."

Creating a Workout Environment

Since these workouts can be complete at home, making sure you have available space to complete exercises is imperative for success. All you really need is a space large enough to spread out a little bit—let's say for example, to complete 10 lunges in a row. While you do not need any equipment, it may be nice to have a yoga mat if you have hard floors like wood or linoleum.

Some prefer a quiet environment to work out or to use a music player to help them focus during their workout. Do whatever puts you in the zone to complete your routine. The point is to try to minimize the space of distractions so you can put in the work to meet your goals.

Summary and Key Points

- Bodyweight Workouts are easy, fast, and are extremely effective for beginners and more seasoned exercisers!
- You can't expect the most comprehensive results without also ensuring your diet falls in line with the changes you want to see on your body!
- Designate a space to complete your workouts in, whether that be your living room or backyard patio.
- Design your space to allow for workout completion depending on space needs and create motivational vibes in the area for inspiration.

Chapter 2: Types of Bodyweight Workouts

Bodyweight workouts can be focused on targeting a specific group of muscles. This chapter will outline bodyweight exercises that target the following areas: arms, legs, chest, back, butt, and abs.

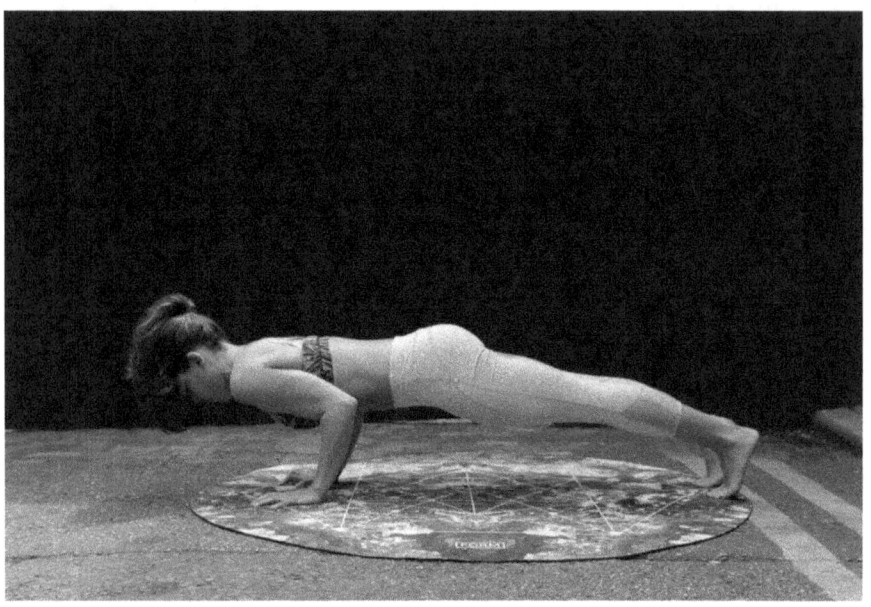

Photo byFormonUnsplash

We all have what we call 'problem areas,' and strength training can be the best and fastest way to target those areas on our bodies that we want to be more toned. Bodyweight Workouts use our own weight to create resistance so we can work on building up muscle on whichever body parts need our attention. Here are some examples of workouts from the before-named areas:

Focus: Arms

- **Tricep Dips**
    - This move helps build up your pectorals, triceps, forearms, and shoulder muscles. Push your chest out and using your arms, lower your body until your elbows are at 90 degrees.

Push back up. Keep your head and chin up during the process.

- **Crab Walk**
    - Get down into a crab position: hands and feet in line with each other and flat on the ground with your chest facing up not down, knees bent, and hips held several inches off the ground. Walk several spaces forward, and then several spaces back.

    - Narrowing your hand placement while completing pushups will engage your core while toning your triceps, pectorals, and shoulders. Start in a pushup position, but instead of your hands lining up with your shoulders, move them in slightly on both sides. Lower your body down, holding yourself up, then push back into the starting position.

Focus: Legs

- **Wall Sit**
    - Set your back up against a stable wall until your knees form a 90-degree angle with the wall. Your head, shoulders, and upper back should be lying flat against the wall, with your weight evenly distributed between both feet.

- **Jump Squat**
    - Standing straight up, keep your arms down by your sides. Squat down normally until your upper thighs are as close to parallel with the floor as they can be. Pressing off with your feet, jump straight up into the air, and as you touch down, go back into the squatting position and start again.

- **Lunges**
    - Starting in a standing position, head and chin up, eyes forward, take a step forward with one leg ensuring your knee is above your ankle. You don't want your other knee to touch the ground. Push back up into standing position and step forward with your opposite leg.

Focus: Chest

- **Incline Pushups**
    - This form is a great modification for those who may just be beginning and are struggling to do a basic pushup. Find some kind of incline in your workout area: a desk, wall, chair, etc. and stand facing the incline with your feet shoulder width apart and feet 1-2 feet back from the wall. Place your hands on either side of the incline and place them slightly wider than your shoulders. Slowly bend the elbows and lower your body toward the incline, pause and push back up—try not to lock your elbows.

- **Traditional Plank**
    - Start off in a pushup position. Instead of lowering yourself and pushing yourself back up, you intend to hold your body in that position. Do not bend your elbows and make sure your feet are not wider than your shoulders. Hold this pose for 10 seconds to begin, and as you begin to master this exercise, work your way up to 30 seconds, 1 minute, etc.

- **Burpees**
    - This move combines several moves into one and can be a killer workout for beginners. Standing straight up, bend down in a position with your hands on the floor supporting your body. Kick back both feet until you are in a plank/pushup position. Quickly jump back on your feet

and spring up, raising your hands to the sky. After lowering your arms, start again by bending back down.

Focus: Back

- **Reverse Snow Angel**
    - Instead of lying on your back like you were about to make a snow angel, flip over and lay face down on the ground. Raise your arms and shoulders off the ground slightly, about two inches, and bring your hands down from your sides up past your head. (If you were standing not laying down you would be raising and lowering your arms in an up and down wing-flapping motion.)

- **Superman**
    - Lie face down on the ground with your toes pointing down under your body. Reach your arms out straight to your sides, and raise both your arms and feet in the air while making sure your torso maintains contact with the ground.

- **Good Mornings aka Hip Hinges**
    - Standing up straight with your hands on your hips and your feet shoulder-width apart, bend forward at your waist until your back is parallel to the ground. Engage your core and bring your torso back up in a straight position. It is important to keep your neck in line with your spine while doing this exercise.

Focus: Butt

- **Fire Hydrants**
    - Start in a modified pushup position—the standard pushup position but with knees and hands on the ground instead of feet and hands on the ground. Raise one leg off the

ground with your knee bent at a 90-degree angle. This move can also be completed with a straight leg for similar results. If you need inspiration, you want to look like a dog who is just about the use a fire hydrant!

- **Leg Kickbacks**
  - Again, start in a modified pushup position. Try to align your shoulders with your knees. Kick one leg back behind you. Make sure you feel the movement in your hips and glutes, not your lower back. Bring your leg back down and switch sides.

- **Glute Bridges**
  - Lay on the ground, flat on your back with your hands by your sides. Place your feet flat on the floor shoulder-width apart. Use your upper back, upper arms, and core to raise your hips up off the ground toward the sky while keeping your feet and arms on the ground. Slowly lower your hips until they are resting back on the ground.

Focus: Abs

- **Side Planks**
  - Lie down on your side on the floor, and place one elbow underneath you so that you are forming a plank on one side. Keeping your elbow underneath your shoulder, push your lower torso up off of the ground so that the only things touching the ground are your right forearm and the side of your right foot or your left forearm and the side of your left foot. Hold the position for ten seconds, release, and then resume the position.

- **Flutter Kicks**
  - Lie on your back on the floor with your arms down by your sides and your heels flat on the ground. Lift your

heels about 6 inches off the ground, and quickly kick your legs up and down. It is easier to complete 10 kicks, rest for 20 seconds, then do another 10 kicks because of how short and quick the kicks are.

- **V-Sit Crunch**
    - Lay flat on your back on the ground with your arms laying above your head. Lift up your legs like you are about to attempt a crunch, but bring your arms up toward your legs at the same time, creating a 'V.' Lower your arms and legs back into the starting position lying down.

Summary and Key Points

- There are many more exercises within each focus category. The ones listed in this book are just suggestions to get you started.
- If you are confused about how to complete an exercise, YouTube has an excellent variety of step-by-step videos.
- It's a great idea to track your repetitions (reps), so you know you started being able to do 10 pushups and now doing 25!

Chapter 3: Planning a Workout Routine That Works For You

Bodyweight workouts are perfect because it can be completed with only some space and your body: no gym or equipment required! An even better bonus to these exercises is that they are so simple to do that they are easily combined to reap even more benefits in the same amount of time.

What to Include In Your Plan

Important aspects of a workout routine include duration, frequency, intensity, and consistency. The Mayo Clinic suggests adults get in about 150 minutes of moderate exercise a week, or 75 minutes of vigorous activity and at least 2 days of strength training: "Moderate aerobic exercise includes activities such as brisk walking, swimming, and mowing the lawn. Vigorous aerobic exercise includes activities such as running and aerobic dancing. Strength training can include the use of weight machines, your own body weight, resistance tubing, resistance paddles in the water, or activities such as rock climbing."

To break this down for you, you should look at workouts with moderate intensity for 3 days a week for 50 minutes each, or 5 days a week for 30 minutes each. It's up to you to decide when you want to schedule your workouts throughout the week, but making sure you start your Mondays with a workout is always a great way to set up your week for success!

How to Stay Dedicated When Your Resolve Falters

A LifeHacker article written by Alan Henry has some great tips on how to motivate yourself to start your routine and how to stick with your routine. Without consistency, you will never see or keep results!

1. Stop Making Excuses
    - Don't be too hard on yourself, we all make mistakes and expect too much from ourselves. Know that failures are an expected part of the journey.

- We all have to start from somewhere—doing something, no matter how small, is better than doing nothing at all!

2. Understand Your Habits
    - "Most people fail in fitness because they never enter a self-sustaining positive feedback loop. To be successful at fitness, it needs to be in the same category of the brain as sleeping, eating, and sex." The key is to find a routine replacement that works for you and gets results for the energy you put into building it into your habits."

    - Starting from zero can cause people to want to give up: "Oftentimes, people are actually lazy because they're out of shape and don't exercise!" It's quite easy for a fit person to tell someone who's having a tough time that they're just lazy, but the reality is that running a mile is much easier for someone who does five every day compared to someone who's been sitting on the couch for most of his life."

3. Find Your "Secret Sauce"
    - "Minimizing and oversimplifying the challenge doesn't help, and while hearing what worked for others can help you figure out things to try, it's almost never going to be exactly what works for you. Look for your own combination of tools, tips, techniques, and advice that will support you and your health and fitness goals."

4. Be Engaged and Stick to Your Plan
    - "Set the bar low and start small. If you're having trouble with working out every day, start with twice or once a week. Whatever it is, start with something you can *definitely* do effortlessly. This is where suggestions like

parking on the far end of the lot and taking the stairs come into play."

- "Whatever you do, make it fun. Whatever you do, enjoy it. Choose something rewarding enough to make you feel good about doing it. If you're having a good time, mistakes feel like learning experiences and challenges to be overcome, not throw-up-your-hands-and-give-up moments."

5. Track Your Victories With Technology
    - "Technology can be a huge benefit to help you see your progress in a way that looking in the mirror won't show you. The goal is to keep that track record, whether it's on a calendar, in an app, or on a website, going unbroken as long as possible. Just remember, quantifying your efforts is just a method to get feedback and track your progress. Your tech should be a means to build better habits, not the habit in itself."

Another great way to keep yourself accountable is by enlisting a friend to work out with you. Even if you don't have the same fitness goals or you don't want to be distracted while you are trying to work out, having someone to be accountable to can really push us to meet our goals. Whether that's a text or a phone call on days you know your friend should be working out, that small reminder may be enough to get them going.

Sample 7-day Routine

After deciding how many days and for how long each day you want to work out, the next step is planning what exercises you will complete in each session. It's not generally recommended that you focus on the same muscle groups two days in a row, although every other day is absolutely fine!

Sunday: Arms

    15 pushups x3

    15 tricep dips x3

    15 lay down pushup x3

    15 walkouts x3

Monday: Legs

    15 jump squats x3

    16 X jumps x3

    15 lunges x3

    24 high knees x3

    10 burpees x3

Tuesday: Rest!

Wednesday: Chest

    10 second plank x3

    15 decline pushups x3

    15 mountain climbers x3

    15 burpees x3

Thursday: Abs

    15 straight leg sit ups x3

    20 ab bikes x3

15 straight leg raises x3

20 side twists

Friday: Rest!

Saturday: Back

15 bridges x3

15 back extensions x3

15 opposite arm/leg raises x3

15 bridges x3

Try to complete all four workouts on each day as fast as you can while resting for up to 30 seconds between each move. If you want to up the intensity, slowly increase the repetitions—a good interval is an increase of 5. Another way to make the workout more intense is to complete the workout as a circuit. If you complete a day's workouts as a circuit, ignore the "repeat 3 times." Instead, you would complete, for example, 15 straight leg sit-ups, 20 ab bikes, 15 straight leg raises, and 20 side twists. Rest for 30 seconds! Repeat starting with 15 straight leg sit-ups. Try to not rest for more than 30 seconds. If you need to when you're just beginning, that's completely okay! Complete one circuit and begin working on adding additional circuits to your workouts.

If you already have a workout routine that you regularly complete, try adding in certain strength training exercises between your cardio workout. Again, slowly build up your repetitions but starting small.

Summary and Key Points

- Plan your workouts into your day with your planner or calendar system. Start small and build your way up to working out 3, 4, or 5 days a week!
- Switch up the muscle groups you focus on to make sure that you see full body results.

- The recommended workouts are only a very small example of workouts within each category to get you started. Research muscle groups you want to target and incorporate those goals into your workout plan.

Chapter 4: How to Make the Most Out of Your Bodyweight Workouts

As touched on in the last chapter regarding circuit workouts, High-Intensity Interval Training is a great way to target multiple muscle groups in one workout and burn more calories. We will also touch on tools that can be used to track your workouts and your progress, as well as an important aspect of ending your workout that is sometimes forgotten but still important: stretching!

High-Intensity Interval Training

According to Bodybuilding.com, "these different body compositions point to the fact that not all cardio is created equal, which is why it's important to choose a form of cardio that meets your goals. A recent study compared participants who did steady-state cardio for 30 minutes three times a week to those who did 20 minutes of high-intensity interval training (HIIT) three times per week. Both groups showed similar weight loss, but the HIIT group showed a 2 percent loss in body fat while the steady-state group lost only 0.3 percent. The HIIT group also gained nearly two pounds of muscle, while the steady-state group lost almost a pound."

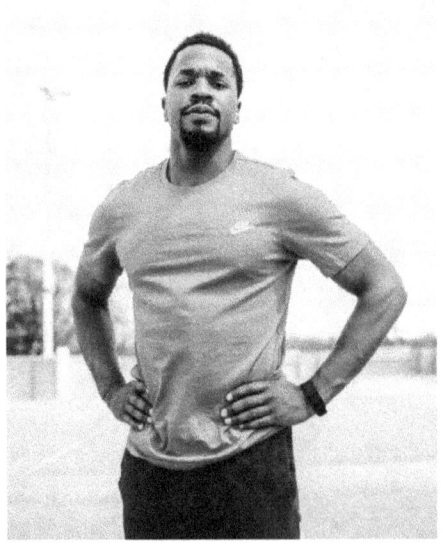

Photo by Autumn Goodman on Unsplash

Progress Can Be Small, But Any Progress is Significant

Tracking your gains is an important part of using body weight workouts. Some people prefer creating their own systems in a notebook or journal, others use electronic devices, and the rest of us prefer to use visual progress indicators.

Writing down when you completed a workout, what exercises you completed, and how many repetitions you completed is a great reminder of your goals and how far you've come on the journey to reach them. Before your next workout, refer back to your last logged workout and see what adjustments you need to make to your workout today to help you be successful.

Technology Can Help Us Keep More Accurate Records

Using a tracking device like a Fitbit watch, hybrid smartwatch, iPhone, or smart shoes, you can track calories burned, distance moved, heart rate, and then have them saved somewhere digitally instead of in a hard copy paper form.

Stretching for Injury Prevention Should Be a Priority

Warming up and then stretching after a workout is an important way to help prevent injuries. Stretch out your arms, legs, back, and any other areas that feel tight.

Key Summary Points

- HIIT workouts are a great way to combine targeting different muscle groups in one workout instead of many.
- Tracking your gains in whichever fashion makes you the most comfortable and that you find the most motivating is highly encouraged!
- Taking 5-15 minutes to stretch after a workout will ease soreness for your workouts in the following days, and will help prevent your muscles from getting injured.

PART 3

Chapter One: Muscle Mass

You have probably heard by now of the many benefits of having more of your body being composed of muscle mass. And yet, I'd venture to guess you still don't know the half of it!

If you're a woman, thirty percent of your body is made up of muscle mass; for men, it's around forty. The bottom line is, we all want more muscle! Muscle gives us that long and lean appearance—with nicely shaped muscles. Muscular people are viewed as healthy people. Obviously, they are also stronger. Too much fat can lead to all kinds of health problems, not to mention all the clothes you have that you can't wear!

There are many, many reasons to desire to build more muscle, but I'll give you the one that is at the top of the list for me: muscle burns fat. That's right! Muscle burns fat not only when you're in the gym or somewhere else, hitting the weights, or doing body resistance training, it does so when you're at rest. That is correct. Muscle eats away at fat while you're lolling on the sofa watching that Sunday afternoon football game.

This is why we love muscle!

Many folks don't do weight training because they think they have to head to the gym. It's a very common myth that it's necessary to use weights in order to add muscle. But it's just that—a myth. You also don't have to purchase a room full of expensive weights, gadgets and other equipment to use to build muscle at home.

I'm going to let you in on a little secret. You can build muscle using just...you. It is true. You can use your own body's resistance against itself to burn fat and build muscle. It's awesome! This way, there are no excuses. You don't have to pay a gym membership, drive yourself there, or even leave the comfort of your own home.

I'm going to give you nine different muscle-building, fat-burning workouts, and we're going to talk—just a little—about a few things you can do in the area of diet. Yes, diet. Not "diet" as in a bad word—like "I feel miserable after eating badly for the last two weeks and I need to go on a diet." Not that sort of talk. We'll simply touch on some of the foods you should be eating and some of the food you shouldn't be if you're genuinely interested in losing some weight.

Before we get into the exercises, let's cover some basics.

How Muscle is Built

Simply put in laymen's terms, when you work out, you essentially damage your muscles. Muscle tissue is broken down. When this process happens, your body gets busy repairing and replacing these damaged tissues. To get just a little technical during this process, the body has a process on the cellular level in which it repairs or replaces the damaged muscle fibers. It fuses these fibers together to form new myofibrils (muscle protein strands). Repaired myofibrils are larger in thickness and are greater in number, thus causing muscle hypertrophy (growth). This process doesn't happen when you are lifting weights, though. It happens afterward when the body is at rest. That's why rest is absolutely a key component to muscle growth. The hard work is only half the process. But fortunately the rest—pun intended—is easy.

Chapter Two: The Upper Body

"Can we please have a moment of silence for all those stuck in traffic on the way to the gym?" —Anonymous

These aren't always the easiest exercises to do—well, actually, exercising isn't exactly easy anyway, so scratch that. The great thing about upper body work is that this is where you will begin to see results first. So, for that reason, doing upper body work can be incredibly rewarding.

1. The Classic Push-Up

Push-ups are super easy, super basic and have been around forever. The reason they've been around forever is that they're also super effective. The key is to perform them correctly. If you don't, they become wasted effort.

The proper way to do push-ups

Get on the ground, belly down. Place your palms on the floor a shoulder width apart or slightly more. Keep your body straight as you push yourself up by extending your arms. Repeat. Make sure that your arms are lifting your body weight, not the muscles on the lower half of your body. Imagine there is a plank of wood on your back starting from your head to your feet. Make sure that your body is as straight as that plank in order to maintain correct body alignment.

How many push-ups?

That depends on the kind of shape you are in when you start. When you begin to do the push-ups, do they feel easy to you? Make sure you are performing the move deliberately—not going too fast that you're using momentum. The first time you try, do as many as you can while still keeping perfect form. Afterward, for your regular sets, do two-thirds that many. So, if you did fifteen but were tired by then and beginning to lose form, use ten as a target for your sets in the beginning.

As you get stronger, make the number higher. You want to continue to be challenged. Some people do as many as one-hundred push-ups per day.

Perhaps that's something you can aim for. For the average beginner, three sets of ten are reasonable.

2. Chair-Dips

This is another upper-body exercise that, while in actuality, you're using your body-weight, you'll still need a chair or a bench or something similar. When I'm out running, there's a square cement planter that has an edge to it, and it works perfectly.

Dips further work the rhomboid muscles in your back and synchronize with push-ups on working your triceps.

- Get a chair/bench or another object capable of supporting your body weight and of a similar height, as explained above. Stand with your back to it. Make sure that the object is sturdy enough to support your entire body weight. Lower yourself and place your palms on the front edge of the bench, fingers pointing forward. Tuck in your elbows to your sides. Maintain this position and walk just your feet slowly in front of you. Your body weight should be resting on your arms now. Deliberately bend your arms and lower yourself. Do this until the floor is parallel to your upper arms. If you're doing it right, you'll feel it in your back and also in your triceps. Simply hold for about a second and return to the starting position.

Do three sets. Determine the number of repetitions per set the exact same way as you did for the push-ups.

3. Diamond Push-Ups

Oh, chicken wings—and not the kind you eat. "Chicken wing" is a common term used to refer to the fat on the back of a person's upper arm as it kind of tends to sag, resulting in an unattractive "flapping in the wind" sort of scenario when you wave your arms. Nobody has time for this, people! Not when there are exercises that will blast those wings if you simply stay consistent. Almost everyone wants tight, toned arms. It's a sexy look, and it's youthful! Tight triceps can actually defy a woman's age.

THE STRENGTH TRAINING PROTOCOL

So don't skimp on the upper body exercises. I'm giving you three here, and all of them work your triceps, but the Diamond Push-Up works it the most of all so if you're only worried about triceps and nothing else, do this one.

- Start in the push-up position, yet instead of having your hands out to the sides, place them in front of you and put them together to create a diamond shape.

- Raise yourself until your legs are straight then lower yourself until you are two inches above the ground. You will feel the burn in those triceps. Embrace the burn! The burn means the move is working.

Choose your number of reps in the same manner with all of the upper body exercises.

Chapter Three: The Core

You must not ignore the importance of core work when it comes to resistance training. Your core muscles are the ones that essentially holds everything else together.

There's a very good chance that, no matter what you're doing, you're using your core. Having a weak core takes the power away from all the rest of your muscles. Your core muscles are also responsible for your balance and stability, which is huge. Your core is not one muscle; it's a complicated interconnected series of muscles which effectively include all of them except your arms and your legs. So, I reiterate. Working your core needs to be an incredibly important part of your exercise routine.

Think about your abs. Everybody seems to be concerned with their abdominal muscles. Many people want those six-pack muscles to show. Some just want to button their favorite jeans without lying on the bed.

There's a common misconception (still) that fat can be "spot-burned." This is simply not true. The general consensus is that fat leaves the body the same way it came on—gradually and kind of all over. Don't get me wrong on this; genetics do play a role in how our bodies store fat. Some people can be perfectly proportioned pretty much everywhere on their bodies and yet have large, unattractive bellies. Those people are still more the exception than the rule.

So, the bottom line is that you cannot target fat-burning. If you really want the fat to leave your body, there are three central areas that will require your attention: diet, cardio, and resistance training. Here we are focusing on the third, and a little later I'm going to give a quick overall snapshot of the importance of combining all three.

I'm going to give you three exercises for your core. This first one, known as a Plank, could actually be used as the only core exercise you do. It is that effective and, especially considering the other exercises you'll be doing with, will touch all the muscles in your core.

Now, remember what we said about abs and fat? Here's something many people simply don't realize. Underneath however much fat we happen to be carrying on our abdominal muscles, we all have a "six-pack." Those are muscles in each of our bodies. What people are trying to do when they say they're going for six-pack abs is burn the layers of fat that cover those muscles. As I said, and much to the sadness of myself and many others, you can't target that weight.

Additionally, I'm not going to include any kind of "sit-ups" in upper body work. They've been proven to not be as effective as other exercises that work the core muscles. Also, I personally think that unless your form is always perfect with a sit-up, you may be putting certain back muscles at risk.

4. Plank

This one is tough, but like I said, with this one exercise and all the many variations you can do with it, you can get those core muscles strong in no time.

- Start with the initial push-up position. Bend your elbows to a right angle. Let your weight rest on your forearms. You might want to get a mat or something soft to use as padding between your arms and the floor. Make sure you have a timer too. The elbows need to be beneath your shoulders directly. Your body should be forming a straight line from head to heels—like a plank. Hold this position for as long as you can without injuring yourself.

Your goal should eventually be to hold it for two minutes. I said eventually for a good reason. Planks are tough. I mean, for a lot of people, a ten-second plank and they're toast. Because so many muscles are used to hold this position, if those muscles aren't strong, it simply can't happen for very long. That's also why planks are such a good indicator of how far you've come. If, when you start it takes all you have to hold a thirty-second plank, I would venture to guess that after a religiously followed routine, within eight weeks you will have worked up to the full two minutes.

Planks are great because there are many variations of them, as well. As you get stronger, try this:

- While in plank position, lift one of your legs as high as you can and hold it there for a count of thirty. Repeat on the other side.

- You can even do a side plank. Lay down on your side with your head propped on your elbow, raise your body in that position and hold it. To increase difficulty with this one, once you are in the up position, try raising your top leg and holding it in that position.

Planks can be thought of as a "Super Move." They literally work all of your muscles. In fact, if one really wanted to, one could do planks only as their resistance training (planks in all their variations, which are many) and achieve the results they're looking for.

5. Reverse Crunch

Okay, so I realize I just got done telling you that sit-ups, which are essentially crunches, are not good for the back muscles. In fact, one physician has said that he has seen no other cause of back injury with the highest rate as traditional crunches.

However, the reverse crunch, despite its name, does not carry the same risks and is excellent at targeting your abdominal muscles.

Here's how to do it:

- Lie down on the floor and fully extend your arms and legs to the sides. Put your palms on the floor. Your arms should actually stay in one place as you perform the entire exercise.

- This is the position you will start from: your legs will be pulled up which will make your thighs form a right angle with the floor. You will want your feet together and also parallel to the floor.
- Move your legs towards your torso. At the same time, roll your pelvis backward. Raise your hips above the floor. The goal is to have your knees touching your chest.

- Hold this position for around a second, then lower back to the starting position.

Again, depending on your ability when you start, gauge the number of reps and sets by how they feel to your body and how hard it is for you to do them at first. Just make sure not to overestimate yourself too much. Muscle soreness from overdoing it is no fun!

6. Mountain Climber

Get into the top of the push-up position. This is the starting position.

> Keeping your back in a straight line, bring your right knee toward your chest. Quickly bring it back to the starting position. Do the same for the left knee. Repeat but speed up the movement, alternating legs quickly as if you were running in place with your hands on the ground.

As far as how many sets, this move isn't exactly structured that way so use seconds to guide you. Try the move until you are really struggling to continue (you'll likely be out of breath) then use two-thirds of those seconds, call it a set, and do three.

Chapter Four: The Lower Body

Working out your lower body is not to be taken lightly or skimped on when doing resistance training. One particular reason for this is because your lower body contains the largest muscle in your entire body: the gluteus maximus.

Not only do most of us like to work out this muscle because it makes us "look" better, it's also a powerhouse. This muscle, along with other gluteal muscles, is one of the great stabilizers of the human body. Keeping these muscles strong can minimize aches and pains in your lower back and hips. The muscles also give you the power you need to do simple things like walk, run, and climb.

So, whenever lower body resistance training is discussed, there are two moves that are practically givens. No, it's not because they're both somewhat torturous—it's because they are effective!

When you're doing your workout, never forget the old adage, "Pain is temporary…(fill in the blank)." Usually, people say, "pain is temporary, quitting lasts forever."

That doesn't exactly apply here, but the point is that if you aren't going to be able to tolerate a little bit of pain, you aren't going to get the same results. Workouts can hurt. Muscles burn. Sometimes by the end of a good workout, you feel like you're about to croak. As far as I'm concerned, those are the very best kind! It means you've really kicked some gluteal maximuses and made some progress for the day. You have to maintain a good attitude if you're going to embark on this journey. Results don't happen overnight, but relatively you will start to see them very quickly (although, in general people who are close to you will notice before you do.) However, nothing is more satisfying than when you do look in the mirror and see results that can't be denied, or when you put on a pair of jeans that has been an eternity since they were last wore and they button easily. It's a powerful feeling.

So, here they come, the not-always-fun but ever-so-productive lower body movements.

7. The Lunge

If you've ever done them, you're probably feeling the burn simply at the thought! When executed correctly, these babies do burn, but they are incredibly effective.

Lunges produce fast results. You will notice that your legs and derriere are more toned and attractive looking. You will feel that you're stronger and you'll notice the difference when you do cardio—assuming you do, of course.

Lunges do not require weights, although weights can be added later on to increase the difficulty as you get into better shape.

Form in lunges is very important. The same is true with all of these exercises. If you're going to put in the effort, you may as well make sure you're doing it right in order to maximize your results.

Following is how to execute a perfect lunge:

- Stand upright and keep your body straight. Pull your shoulders back and relax your chin. Keep your chin pointed forward, don't look down. Make sure the muscles in your core are tight and engaged.
- If it helps you with balance, you can use something you have on hand, like, say, a broom. Hold it crossways in front of you and let it lightly rest on your shoulders.
- Pick a leg. Step forward using that leg. Lower your hips until both your knees are forming a right angle. Make sure that your lowered knee isn't touching the floor and that your forward knee is directly above your angle and not too far forward. Make sure that your weight is in your heels as you push yourself back up to the starting position.
- When you do push back up to the starting position, really place extra emphasis on engaging your gluteus maximus. Deliberately use the strength in that muscle to push yourself upright.

Now. Repeat. How many times? I recommend starting with three sets of ten perfectly executed lunges. If you don't feel "the burn" add a couple, or go ahead and use a barbell if you have one and put some weight on it. You can even do lunges in reverse, to vary things up.

8. Squat

Ah, the squat. If you haven't done them, you've probably heard of them if you have any friends at all who work out. Like lunges, they are simple, easy to execute, and incredibly effective at increasing muscle mask and making you stronger.

Also, like lunges, there are quite a few variations to squats that you can use as you get more fit. For now, of course, we'll focus on the simple squat. Again, form is super important.

- Stand with your feet at least shoulder-width apart. If you feel more comfortable, it's okay to place your feet a bit wider apart. As you stand, you should focus on having your weight on your heels. Extend your arms straight out. The first thing you'll do is thrust your hips back slightly as though you are about to take a seat. Then, lower yourself down like that as if you are actually about to sit down. You'll want to go as low as you can. The goal is to make your knees bent so that your legs are parallel to the floor, again almost if you were sitting in a chair. Control your knees so they don't move forward over your feet.
- The next step is simply to stand up, and when you are coming upright, squeeze your glutes at the top of the movement. So, essentially, squats are like sitting in an invisible chair, then standing up using your glutes to propel you. Very easy but super effective!

9. The Bridge

The bridge is another great one for strengthening your glutes and legs. Remember, before you even see the results of these exercises, you'll be stronger for doing them. And, if you eat right and take in enough protein (building blocks for muscle) you will increase the size of your muscle and consequently burn fat. So when you're doing these not-so-fun-at-the-time moves, keep that in mind!

- Here's how to do a bridge: Lie on the floor, flat as a pancake. Place your hands on your sides and bend your knees. Your feet should be about shoulder-width apart. Lift your hips off the floor, using your heels to push. Keep your back straight while doing this! Hold the position for a second and squeeze those glutes.
- Slowly lower back to the position you started from.

For the number of reps, use the method we discussed previously. The first time you try the exercise, go until you really feel the burn—until it's very tough to continue or until you would not be able to. However many reps that is (say it's fifteen) subtract one-third of that number and start from there.

For variety, this exercise can be performed with one leg at a time.

Chapter Five: Putting it all Together

People have different preferences in how they like to work out. To see good results from strength training, you need to work each muscle group no less than two times per week. Three times is fine and you may see faster results that way. Depending on what you want to accomplish, generally, three times is enough.

The idea is to give each muscle group a rest day in between your workouts. So people go about the entire construct differently. Some like to work their entire body in one session, then rest for a day or two and do it again, up to three times a week.

Others prefer to break the muscle group workouts up. Legs one day, arms the next, core the next, like that.

In my opinion and in consideration of the research I've done, any of the above-mentioned ways to go about it will be just as effective as another. Of course, the most important component is that it gets done.

I'd like to take a moment at the time to talk about cardiovascular workouts. I know, I know, boo, hiss. A lot of people really aren't that big on cardio. However, there's a lot to be said for a good cardio sweat session. For one thing, cardiovascular exercise improves the health of our heart and lungs. That alone should be reason enough to work some in. Also, this type of exercise, depending on the type you choose, can burn an awful lot of calories. Remember, any calories burned will contribute to that sleek, muscular look. For the muscles to come out, the fat has to come off.

Cardiovascular exercise has also been proven to affect our moods in a positive way (the same can be said for weight training.)

The best, most well-rounded exercise plans include a mixture of both. Supposing you hate cardio, you will do yourself no harm by keeping it to a minimum. The general recommendation right now is to get thirty minutes of cardio on "most" days of the week.

Given that, as an example, you could do your weights on Monday, cardio Tuesday, weights Wednesday, Cardio Thursday, weights Friday and guess what? Take the weekend off!

This is just one example of how this can all be done. You can be as creative as you want to be or as you need to be to get around a work schedule.

You could do, for instance, cardio in the morning and resistance training at night. You could work in all or part of your resistance training during your lunch hour at work.

There are no limits to the options available, so that simply means *no excuses*.

No equipment or anything fancy is required for the cardio portion either. Walking is cardio. Just walk fast enough to get your heart rate up, break a sweat and breathe a little heavy. Increase intensity as your fitness level improves.

Here's a sample plan, if you need one. I'm going to use ten reps as a standard while performing the strength training for the sake of simplicity.

Monday Morning Before Work:

Three sets of ten of each of the following:

- Push-ups
- Chair-Dips
- Diamond Push-ups

Honestly, this should take you no more than ten minutes.

Monday Lunch:

- Walk for thirty minutes

Monday Evening:

Perform three sets of the following:

- Squats
- Lunges
- Bridges
- Planks
- Mountain Climber
- Reverse Crunch

Starting out, repeat this same routine on Wednesdays and Fridays. Try this for a few weeks (or another plan of your own design) and see how it works with your schedule.

On the days that you don't walk for thirty-minutes on your lunch, per your official "schedule," do it anyway. If not that, jump on the trampoline with your little ones at night for half an hour. Ride your bike. Swim. Ski if you live near snow and/or if it's wintertime. Snow Show. Or...head to the gym. Do the elliptical or the stair-climber for half of an hour. It's really not hard to get in the minimum amount of cardio and depending on your goals, and who says you have to stop with the minimum?

If you stick to this program, you're going to see some results and you'll see them pretty quickly.

Here's another tip: throw away your scale. Okay, well you don't have to throw it away. I just don't recommend weighing yourself all the time. It could discourage you in fact, for the simple reason that muscle actually does weigh more than fat. You might gain in the beginning, and no one wants to start a workout program only to see the numbers on the scale go up. No way! Instead of worrying about the scale, judge your progress by —most importantly—how you feel, and as for changes in your body, you can always take some initial measurements and then re-measure once a week. What has always worked best for me is simply to gauge how my clothes fit. That's the biggest tell of all. I have a pair of jean shorts I'm wearing right now. A couple of months ago I couldn't get them to even think about zipping! That's the only kind of progress I need. To me, numbers on the scale don't mean a whole lot.

Chapter Six: On Your Diet

It wouldn't be right to talk about gaining muscle and losing fat without talking a bit about diet.

I'm not going to go overboard but there are a few things I'd like to touch on.

First off, as I previously spoke about at the end of chapter four—the scale—I forgot to mention another reason I don't care to use them. Most of them have a tendency to fluctuate as much as five pounds in less than twenty-four hours. In other words, if I'm going by the scale, I often will have "gained" five pounds from when I got up to when it's time for bed.

Not cool.

Not possible, either. Our bodies are made up of an estimated sixty-five percent water. It is normal for the amount of water in our bodies to fluctuate all the time. Losing water weight does not equate to losing fat. However, while we are trying to lose weight, and while we're working out, it is especially important to keep our bodies hydrated.

There are as many theories on the web as you could click on about how much water to drink, but for questions like these, I like to refer to the Mayo Clinic website, because I know that the information they put out there has been thoroughly researched. What follows is their advice on water intake:

Every single day, you lose water by breathing, sweating, urinating, and pooping. To function properly, your body's water must be replenished through the consumption of food and beverages.

The average healthy man who lives in a temperate climate needs 15.5 cups or 3.7 liters of fluids every day, and the average healthy woman living in the same place needs 11.5 cups or 2.7 liters every day.

This is about what I do for myself in a normal day and it seems to work. Regardless, don't skimp on the water.

There's another important factor when it comes to building muscle and that is protein. If you are serious about adding some muscle mass, you're going to need to eat your protein. That doesn't mean it has to be meat; there are plenty of non-meat options for protein intake. Of course, if you are a vegetarian you already know that.

Another little tip: your body needs fat to lose fat. Sounds strange, doesn't it? But if your body is starved of nutrients, it will begin to hold on to everything it has instinctually, and as a result, you won't see any weight loss.

There are a million types of "diets" out there, and this is not a book about diets so I'm not going to delve into them. If I were going to say anything at all about your diet (and don't get me wrong, your diet IS important,) I would say two words: eat clean.

What does that mean? Since clean is the opposite of dirty, in this case, think dirty equals "processed."

Do your body a giant favor and stay away from processed foods! Eat foods that are as "close" to the earth as you can.

- Lean proteins (including fish and non-meat proteins)
- Tons—and I do really mean tons—of vegetables
- Lean fat (avocado, almonds, coconut oil)
- Dairy (full-fat; eat sparingly)
- Fruits (sparingly)

It's that simple. No "TV Dinners." No boxes of macaroni and cheese, please. Nothing that has a "bunch" of ingredients, many of which you aren't even familiar with. Those are bad. Leave them in the store.

If you have a sweet tooth, indulge it, but rarely, and even a sweet tooth can be indulged in a healthy manner. There's nothing wrong with eating some strawberries topped with full fat whipped cream. Yummy!

Well, there you have it. You really are set. Everything is explained and condensed for you.

Start your weight training and your cardio, eat clean, drink your water and reap the rewards.

Go get 'em!

PART 4

PART 4.1

What Is Fasting and Why You Should Do It

Chapter 1: What Is Fasting?

Introduction to Fasting

Latest Research and Studies about Fasting

In a research published by the Springer Journal, it was found that fasting helps fight against obesity. The study, led by Kyoung Han Kim and Yun Hye Kim, was aimed at tracking the effects of fasting on fat cells. They put a group of mice into a four-month period of intermittent fasts, where the mice were fed for two days, followed by a day of fasting. In the end, the group of fasting mice was found to weigh less than the non-fasting mice, even though all of them had consumed exact quantities of food. The group of fasting mice had registered a drop in the fat buildup around fat cells. The explanation was that the fat had been converted into energy when glucose was insufficient. (www.sciencedaily.com/releases/2017/10/171017110041.htm)

In November 2017, Harvard researchers established that fasting can induce a long life, as well as minimize aging effects. It was found that fasting revitalizes mitochondria. Mitochondria are the organelles that act as body power plants. In this replenished state, mitochondria optimize physiological functions, in effect slowing down the aging process. Fasting also promotes low blood glucose levels, which improves skin clarity and boosts the immune system. (https://newatlas.com/fasting-increase-lifespan-mitochondria-harvard/52058/)

Sebastian Brandhorst, a researcher based at the University of Southern California, found out that fasting has a positive impact on brain health. Fasting induces low blood sugar levels, causing the liver to produce ketone bodies that pass on to the brain in place of sugars. Ketone bodies are much more stable and efficient energy sources than glucose. Researchers from the same university have posited that fasting minimizes chances of coming down with diabetes and other degenerative diseases. Moreover, they discovered that fasting induces low production of the IGF-1 hormone, which is a catalyst in aging and spread of disease. (https://www.cnbc.com/2017/10/20/science-diet-fasting-may-be-more-important-than-just-eating-less.html)

Biological Effects of Fasting

- **Cleanses the body**

Our bodies harbor an endless count of toxins, and these toxins announce their presence through symptoms like low energy, infections, allergies, terrible moods, bloating, confusion, and so on.

Eliminating toxins from your body will do you a world of good in the sense that your body will upgrade and start functioning optimally. There are many ways to cleanse your body: hydrotherapy, meditation, organic diets, herbs, yoga, etc.

But one of the most effective ways of cleansing your body is through fasting. When you go on a fast, you allow the body to channel the energy that would have been used for digestion into flushing out toxins.

- **Improves heart health**

Studies show that people who undertake regular fasts are less likely to contract coronary infections. Fasting fights against obesity, and obesity is a recipe for heart disease. It purifies the blood too, in that sense augmenting the flow of blood around the body.

- **Improves the immune system**

Fasting rids the body of toxins and radicals, thus boosting the body's immune system and minimizes the chances of coming down with degenerative diseases like cancer. Fasting reduces inflammation as well.

- **Improves bowel movement**

One of the problems of consuming food on the regular is that the food sort of clogs up your stomach, causing indigestion. You might go for days without visiting the bathroom to perform number two. But when you fast, your body resources won't be bogged down by loads of undigested foods, and so your bowel movement will be seamless. Also, fasting promotes healthy gut bacteria.

- **Induces alertness**

When your stomach is full because of combined undigested foods (i.e., "garbage"), you are more likely to experience brain-fog. You won't have any concentration on the tasks at hand. You will just sit around and laze the hours away, belching and spitting. But when you fast, your mind will be clear so it will be easy to cultivate focus.

Treating Fasting as a Lifestyle Choice

When you perform a simple Google search for the word "fasting," millions of results come up. Fasting is slowly becoming a mainstream subject. This is mostly because of the research-backed evidence that has been published by many reputable publications listing down the various benefits of fasting such as improved brain health, increased production of the human growth hormone, a stronger immune system, heart health, and weight loss—thus its appeal to health-conscious people as a catalyst for their health goals.

Taking up fasting as a lifestyle choice will see you go without food for anywhere from a couple of hours to days. But before you get into it, you'd do yourself a world of good to first obtain clearance from a physician, certifying that your body is ready, because not everyone is made for it. For instance, the symptoms of illnesses such as cancer may worsen after a long stretch of food deprivation. So people with degenerative diseases such as cancer should consider getting professional help or staying away altogether. Pregnant women, malnourished people, and children are advised to stay clear too.

The first thing you must do is to establish your fasting routine. For instance, you may choose to skip breakfast, making lunch your first meal of the day. Go at it with consistency. Also, you may decide to space your meals over some hours; so that when the set hours elapse, you reach your eating window, and then go back to fasting. The real challenge is staying committed. You will find that it will be difficult to break the cycle of eating that your body had been accustomed to, but when you persevere; your body will, of course, adjust to your new habit. If you decide to go for days without food, the results will be far pronounced, but please remember to hydrate your body constantly to flush out toxins.

Summary

Fasting is the willing abstinence from food over a period of time with the goal of improving your life. Conventionally, fasting has been tied to religious practices, but a new school of thought has emerged to proclaim the health benefits of fasting—particularly, weight loss. When you go into a fast, you create a caloric deficit, which triggers the body to convert its fat stores into energy. Numerous studies by mainstream health organizations have been done on fasting, and researchers have established that fasting has a host of advantages like improved motor skills, cognition, and moods. Some of the biological effects of fasting include improved bowel movement, immune system, and heart health. If you are starting out with fasting, you must create a routine and abide by it. Not everyone is fit to practice fasting. Some of the people advised to stay away from the practice include extremely sick people, pregnant women, the malnourished, and children. If you undertake a prolonged fast, you should hydrate your body constantly.

Chapter 2: Obesity and the Standard American Diet

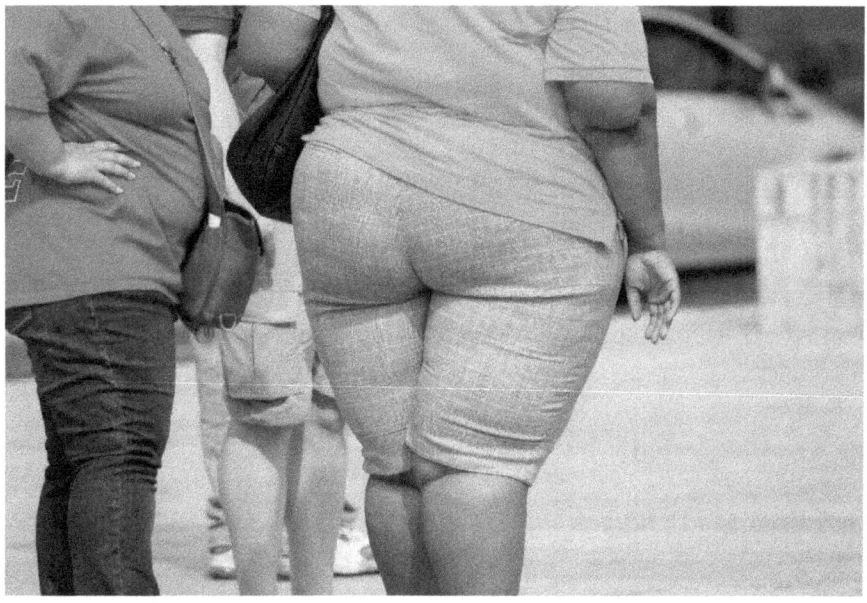

The Obesity Epidemic

We are killing ourselves with nothing more than a spoon and a fork. In 2017, obesity claimed more lives than car accidents, terrorism, and Alzheimer's combined. And the numbers are climbing at a jaw-dropping rate. Obesity has become a crisis that we cannot afford to ignore anymore.

You'd be mistaken to think that obesity is a crisis in first-world economies alone. Even developing nations are experiencing an upsurge of obese citizens. Here comes the big question: what is the **main** force behind this epidemic?

According to new research published in the New England Journal of Medicine, excessive caloric intake and lack of exercise are to blame.

Most American fast food chains have now become global. Fast foods, which are particularly calorie-laden, appeal to a lot of people across the world because of their low prices and taste. So, most people get hooked on the fast food diet and slowly begin the plunge into obesity.

The United States recognizes obesity as a health crisis and lawmakers have petitioned for tax increment on fast foods and sugary drinks, except that for a person who's addicted to fast foods, it would take a lot more than a price increase to discourage their food addiction. It would take a total lifestyle change.

Exercising alone won't help you; no matter how powerful your reps may be, or leg lifts or anything else you try in the gym, nothing can save you from a terrible diet.

And here's the complete shocker; the rate of childhood obesity has surpassed adulthood obesity; a terrible, terrible situation considering that childhood obesity almost always leads to heart complications in adult life.

Why Are We So Fat?

- **Poor food choices**

The number one reason why we are so fat is our poor choice of food. We eat too much of the wrong food, and most of it is not expended, so it becomes stored up as fat.

- **Bad genetics**

It's true that some people are genetically predisposed to gain more weight. Their genetics have wired them to convey abnormal hunger signals, so their bodies pressure them into consuming much more food.

- **Lack of strenuous activities**

Our modern-day lives involve only light physical tasks. Contrast that with the era of the dawn of humanity. Back then people would use up a lot of energy to perform physical activities and survive in unforgiving habitats. Most of the food they consumed would be actually utilized. But today, thanks to our technological advancement, we have been spared from taking part in laborious activities. This makes it hard to use up the energy from food, and the body opts to store it as fat.

- **Psychological issues**

Some of us react to bad moods by indulging in food—in particular, high-calorie fast foods—because the taste of fast foods appeals to our unstable emotions. When we fall in the habit of rewarding our bad moods or depression with binge eating, we unsuspectingly fall into the trap of food addiction, to the point of getting depressed when we fail to binge eat, kicking off our journey into obesity.

- **The endocrine system**

The thyroid's hormones play a critical role in the metabolic rate of a person. Ideally, a strong endocrine system means a high metabolic rate. And so, individuals who have a weakened endocrine system are much more likely to develop obesity.

The Problem with Calories

Calories are the basic units for quantifying the energy in the food we consume. A healthy man needs a daily dose of around 2500 calories to function optimally, and a woman needs 2000 calories.

This caloric target should be met through the consumption of various foods containing minerals, vitamins, antioxidants, fiber, and other important elements, and this is not hard at all to achieve if you adhere to the old-fashioned "traditional diet."

But the challenge is that nowadays, we have many foods with a high caloric count, and yet they hardly fill us up! For instance, fries, milkshake, and a burger make up nearly 2000 calories! You can see how easy it'd be to surpass the caloric limit by indulging in fast food.

When we consume more calories than we burn, our bodies store up the excess calories as fat, and as this process repeats itself over time, the fat has a compounding effect that leads to weight gain.

The only way to make your weight stable is through balancing out the energy you consume with the energy you expend. But for someone who suffers from obesity, if they'd like to have a normal weight, they must create a caloric deficit, and fasting is the surefire practice of creating such a deficit.

Besides checking your caloric intake, you might also consider improving your endocrine system and the efficiency of both your kidney and liver, because they have a direct impact on how the body burns calories. When you buy food products, always find out their caloric count to assess how well they'll fit within your daily caloric needs.

The American Diet

In a 2016 lifestyle survey, most Americans admitted that it is not easy to keep their diet clean and healthy. This isn't surprising, especially when you consider the fact that the average American consumes more than 20 pounds of sweeteners each year. The over-emphasis of sugar and fat in the American diet is the leading cause of obesity in Americans. Illnesses triggered by obesity long started marching into our homes. What we have now is a crisis. But let's find out the exact types of foods that Americans like to feast on (we are big on consuming, it's no secret).

As a melting point of cultures drawn from various parts of the world, it's kind of difficult to say exactly what the all-American favorite foods are. But the United States Department of Agriculture might shine some light on this. It listed down desserts, bread, chicken, soda, and alcohol, as the top five sources of calories among Americans. As you can see, the sugar intake is impossibly high. Interestingly, the US Department of Agriculture also noted that Americans aren't big on fruits.

Pizza may qualify as the all-time favorite snack of America, followed closely by burgers and other fast food. There is a reason why most fast food restaurants are successful in America and throughout the world.

It has also been established that the average American drinks about a gallon of soda every week. Even drinks that are supposed to have a low-calorie count end up being calorie-bombs because of the doctoring that takes place. For instance, black coffee is low on calorie, but not so if it has milk and ice cream and sugar all over it.

Summary

The first-world economies are not alone in facing the crisis of obesity. It has emerged that people in poor countries are battling obesity too. Obesity-related deaths are on the rise. In 2017, the figures were especially shocking, for they'd surpassed the death count of terrorist attacks, accidents, and Alzheimer's combined. One of the corrective measures that the US government is considering to undertake is tax increment on sugars. The chief reason why we are so fat is our poor diets. Our foods are laden with sugars and fats, and it doesn't help that our lifestyles allow us to expend only a small amount of energy, which leads to fat accumulation and consequent weight gain. The average man requires around 2500 calories for his body to act optimally whereas the average woman requires 2000 calories. The top five daily sources of calories for Americans include desserts, bread, chicken, soda, and alcohol.

Chapter 3: Benefits of Fasting

- **Improved Insulin Sensitivity**

Insulin sensitivity refers to how positively or negatively your body cells respond to insulin. If you have a high insulin sensitivity, you will need less amount of insulin to convert the sugars in your blood into energy, whereas someone with low insulin sensitivity would need a significantly larger amount of insulin.

Low insulin sensitivity is characterized by increased blood sugar levels. In other words, the insulin produced by the body is underutilized when converting sugars into energy. Low insulin sensitivity may make you vulnerable to ailments such as cancer, heart disease, type 2 diabetes, stroke, and dementia.

Ailments and bad moods are the general causes of low insulin sensitivity. However, high insulin sensitivity is restored once the ailments and bad moods are over.

Fasting is shown to have a positive effect on insulin sensitivity, enhancing your body to use small amounts of insulin to convert blood sugar into energy.

Improved insulin sensitivity has a great impact on health: leveling up physiological functions and fighting off common symptoms of ailments like lightheadedness and lethargy.

To increase insulin sensitivity, here are some of the best practices: perform physical activities, lose weight, consume foods that are high in fiber and low in Glycemic load, improve your moods and alleviate depressed feelings, and finally, make sure to improve the quality of your sleep.

The rate of insulin sensitivity is also heavily dependent on lifestyle changes. For instance, if you take up sports and exercise, insulin sensitivity goes up, but if you become lazy and inactive, it goes down.

- **Increased Leptin Sensitivity**

Leptin is the hormone that determines whether you're experiencing hunger or full. This hormone plays a critical role in weight loss and health management, and if your body grows insensitive to it, you become susceptible to some ailments. Understanding the role of leptin in your body is critical as it goes into helping you improve your health regimen.

Whenever this hormone is secreted by the fat cells, the brain takes notice, and it tries to determine whether you are in need of food or are actually full. Leptin needs to work as normally as possible else you will receive an inaccurate signal that will cause you to either overfeed or starve yourself.

Low leptin sensitivity induces obesity. This condition is normally witnessed in people with high levels of insulin. The excessive sugars in blood are carried off by insulin into fat cells, but when there is an insulin overload, a communication crash is triggered between fat cells and the brain. This condition induces low leptin sensitivity. When this happens, your brain is unable to tell the exact amount of leptin in your blood, and as such it misleads you. Low leptin sensitivity causes the brain to continue sending out the hunger signal even after you are full. This causes you to eat more than you should and, given time, leads to chronic weight gain.

Fasting has been shown to increase leptin sensitivity, a state that allows the brain to be precise in determining blood leptin quantities, and ensures that the accurate signal is transmitted to control your eating habits.

- **Normalized Ghrelin Levels**

Known as the "hunger hormone," ghrelin is instrumental in regulating both appetite and the rate of energy distribution into body cells.

Increased levels of ghrelin cause the brain to trigger hunger pangs and secrete gastric acids as the body anticipates you to consume food.

It is also important to note that both ghrelin and leptin receptors are located on the same group of brain cells, even though these hormones play contrasting roles, i.e., ghrelin being the hunger hormone, and leptin the satiety hormone.

The primary role of ghrelin is to increase appetite and see to it that the body has a larger fat reservoir. So, high ghrelin levels in your blood will result in you wanting to eat more food and, in some cases, particular foods like cake or fries or chocolate.

People who have low ghrelin levels will not eat enough amounts of food and are thus vulnerable to diseases caused by underfeeding. As a corrective measure, such people should receive shots of ghrelin to restore accurate hunger signals in their bodies.

Studies show that obese people suffer from a disconnection between their brains and ghrelin cells, so the blood ghrelin levels go through the roof, which makes these people be in a state of perpetual hunger. So, these obese people respond to their hunger pangs by indulging in their foods of choice, and thus the chronic weight gain becomes hard to manage.

It has been proven that fasting has a positive effect on ghrelin levels. Fasting streamlines the faulty communication between the brain receptors and ghrelin cells. When this is corrected, the brain starts to send out accurate hunger signals, discouraging you from eating more than you should.

- **Increased Lifespan And Slow Aging**

A study by Harvard researchers demonstrated that intermittent fasting led to an increased lifespan and the slowing down of the aging process. These findings were largely hinged on the cell-replenishing effects of fasting and flushing out of toxins.

The average person puts their digestive system under constant load because they're only a short moment away from their next meal. And given the fact that most foods are bacteria-laden, the immune system becomes strained with all the wars that it must be involved in. This makes the body cells prone to accelerated demise. But what happens when you go on a fast?

The energy that would have previously gone into digesting food is used to flush out toxins from the body instead. Also, it has been observed that body cells are strengthened during a fast, which makes physiological functions a bit more robust.

Fasting also enhances the creation of new neural pathways and regeneration of brain cells. This goes towards optimizing the functions of your brain. And, as we know, an energetic brain makes for a "youthful" life.

When you are on a fast, the blood sugar levels are generally down. The skin responds favorably to low blood sugar levels by improving elasticity and keeping wrinkles at bay. A high blood sugar level is notorious for making you ashy and wrinkly.

Fasting may increase your lifespan even from an indirect perspective. For instance, fasting may develop your sense of self-control, improve your discipline, and even increase your creativity. These immaterial resources are very necessary for surviving in the real world.

- **Improved Brain Function**

Fasting triggers the body to destroy its weak cells in a process known as autophagy. One of the main benefits of autophagy is reducing inflammation. Also, autophagy makes way for new and healthy body cells. Autophagy promotes neurogenesis, which is the creation of new brain cells.

Fasting allows the body to deplete the sugars in the blood, and since the body must continue to operate lest it shuts down, the body turns to an alternative energy source: fats. Through the aid of the liver, ketone bodies are produced to supply energy to the brain. Ketone bodies are a much cleaner and reliable source of energy than carbohydrates. Ketone bodies are known to tone down the effects of inflammatory diseases like arthritis.

Fasting promotes high insulin sensitivity. In this way, the body uses less insulin to convert sugars into energy. High insulin sensitivity means that the body will send out accurate signals when it comes to informing the host of either hunger or satiation.

Fasting enhances the production of BDNF (Brain-Derived Neurotrophic Factor), which a plays a critical part in improving neuroplasticity. And thus more resources are committed to the functions of the brain. BDNF is responsible for augmenting areas like memory, learning, and emotions.

Fasting supercharges your mind. It does so through facilitating the creation of new mitochondria. And since mitochondria are the power plants of our bodies, the energy output goes up. This increase in energy and resources causes the brain to function at a much higher level and yields perfect results.

- **Improved Strength And Agility**

When you think of a person that is considered strong and agile, your mind might conceive a well-muscled individual with veins bulging out their neck. Strength and agility come down to practice and more practice. The easiest way to develop agility and strength is obviously through physical training and sticking to a routine until your body adapts.

You must practice every day to be as strong and agile as you'd want to be. Also, you must take particular care over your dietary habits. Professional athletes stick to a diet that has been approved by their doctors for a reason. When it comes to developing strength and agility, nothing matches the combination of exercise and a flawless diet.

But besides fulfilling these two requirements, fasting, too, has its place. Did you know that you can amplify your strength and agility through fasting?

Fasting provokes the body to secrete the Human Growth Hormone. This hormone enhances organ development and even muscle growth. So when you fast, the HGH hormone might be secreted, and it will amplify the effects of your exercise and diet regimen, making you many times stronger and agile.

Fasting will promote the renewal of your body cells and thus lessen the effects of inflammation. When you perform physical exercises, you're basically injuring and damaging your body cells. So, when you fast, you'll allow your body to destroy its weak cells, and make room for new body cells through biogenesis.

Additionally, fasting will go a long way toward improving your motor skills, making you walk with the grace of a cat, with your body parts flexible.

- **Improved Immune System**

The immune system is responsible for defending your body against organisms that are disease vectors. When a foreign organism enters your body, and the body considers it harmful, the immune system immediately comes into action.

Some of the methods suggested for improving the immune system include having a balanced diet, quality sleep, improving your mental health, and taking physical exercises.

Fasting is an understated method of boosting your immune system.

In a research conducted by scientists at the University of Southern California, it emerged that fasting enhanced the rejuvenation of the immune system. Specifically, new white blood cells were formed, strengthening the body's defense system.

The regeneration of the immune system is especially beneficial to people who have a weak body defense mechanism—namely, the elderly, and the sick. This could probably be the reason why an animal in the wild responds to illness by abstaining from food.

In the same study, it was shown that there is a direct correlation between fasting and diminished radical elements in the body. Cell biogenesis was responsible for eradicating inflammation. And moreover, a replenished immune system discouraged the growth of cancer cells.

Depending on how long you observe a fast, the body will, at one point, run out of sugars, and then it will turn to your fat reservoirs to provide energy for its many physiological functions. Fats make for a much cleaner and stable and resourceful energy source than sugars ever will.

So, relying on this fat-energy, the immune system tends to function at a most optimal level.

- **Optimized Physiological Functions**

These are some of the body's physiological functions: sweating, bowel movement, temperature regulation, urinating, and stimuli response.

In a healthy person, all physiological functions should be seamless, but that cannot be said for most of us because our lifestyles get in the way.

So, the next time you rush to the bathroom intending to take a number two only to wind up spending half an hour there, you might want to take a close look at what you are eating.

Fasting is a great method of optimizing your physiological functions. When you observe a normal eating schedule, your body is under constant strain to keep digesting food—a resource-intensive process. But when you go on a fast, the energy that would have been used for digesting food will now be channeled into other critical functions. For instance, the body may now start ridding itself of radicals that promote indigestion, or amp up the blood circulation system, or even devote energy toward enhancing mental clarity, with the result being optimized physiological functions.

With more resources freed up from the strain of digestion, physiological processes will continue seamlessly, and once the glycogen in the blood is over, the body will continue to power physiological functions with energy acquired from fat cells.

The cellular repair benefits attached to fasting enables your body to perform its functions way better. Fasting reduces oxidative stress, which is a key accelerator of aging. In this way, fasting helps restore the youthfulness of your body cells, and the cells are very much optimized for performance.

- **Improved Cardiovascular Health**

When we talk about cardiovascular health, we are essentially talking about the state of the heart, and specifically, its performance in blood circulation.

Factors that improve the condition of your heart include a balanced diet, improved emotional and mental state, quality sleep, and living in a good environment. When cardiovascular health is compromised, it might lead to fatal consequences.

Researchers have long established that fasting improves cardiovascular health.

One of the outcomes of fasting is cholesterol reduction. The lesser cholesterol you have in your blood, the more seamless the movement of blood through your body. Complications are minimal or nonexistent. Thus your heart will be in a great condition.

Fasting also plays a critical role in toning down diabetes. The average diabetic tends to have low insulin sensitivity. For that reason, they need more insulin than is necessary to convert sugars into energy. It puts a strain on body organs and especially the pancreas. This might cause a trickle-down complication that goes back to the heart.

When the body enters fasting mode, it starts using up the stored energy to fulfill other important physiological functions such as blood circulation, in this way boosting the effectiveness of the heart.

Fasting helps you tap into your "higher state." The effects of matured spiritual energy and peaceful inner self cannot be gainsaid. Someone who's at peace with both himself and the universe is bound to develop a very healthy heart, as opposed to one who's constantly bitter, and one who feels as though he's drowning in a bottomless pit.

- **Low Blood Pressure**

People who have a high blood pressure are at risk of damaging not only their heart but their arteries too. When the pressure of the blood flowing in your arteries is high over a long period of time, it is bound to damage the cells of your arteries, and in the worst case scenario, it might trigger a rupture, and cause internal bleeding. High blood pressure puts you at risk of heart failure. Your heart might overwork itself and slowly start wearing out, eventually grinding to a halt.

In people with high blood pressure, a bigger-than-normal left heart is common, and the explanation is that their left heart struggles to maintain the cardiovascular output. So it starts bulking up and eventually creates a disrupting effect on your paired organ. Another risk associated with high blood pressure is coronary disease. This ailment causes your arteries to thin out to the point that it becomes a struggle for blood to flow into your heart. The dangers of coronary disease include arrhythmia, heart failure, and chest pain.

I started by mentioning the risks of high blood pressure because observing a fast normalizes your blood pressure. With a normal blood pressure, you can reverse these risks. Also, normal blood pressure improves the sensitivity of various hormones like ghrelin and leptin, eliminating the communication gap between brain receptors and body cells.

The low blood pressure induced by fasting causes you to have improved motor skills. It is common to hear people admit that fasting makes them feel light and flexible.

- **Decreased Inflammation**

Inflammation is an indication that the body is fighting against an infectious organism. It causes the affected parts to appear red and swollen.

Many diseases that plague us today are rooted in inflammation, and by the look of things, inflammation will be stuck with us for longer than we imagine.

The role of inflammation in mental health cannot be understated. Inflammation is to blame for bad moods, depression, and social anxiety.

The good news though is that fasting can reduce inflammation. Fasting has been shown to be effective in treating mental problems that are rooted in inflammation and as well as safeguarding neural pathways.

Individuals who have incorporated fasting into their lives are much less likely to suffer breakdowns and bad moods than people who don't fast at all.

Asthma, a lung infection, also has an inflammatory background. What's interesting is that fasting alleviates the symptoms of asthma.

The level of hormone sensitivity determines absorption rates of various elements into body cells. For instance, low insulin sensitivity worsens the rate of conversion of sugar into energy. Fasting improves insulin sensitivity, and thus more sugars can be converted into energy.

Fasting enhances the brain to form new pathways when new information is discovered. In this way, your memory power receives a boost, and you are better placed to handle stress and bad thoughts.

Fasting is very efficient in alleviating gut inflammation. Constant fasting promotes healthy gut flora which makes for great bowel movements.

Fasting is a great means of reducing heart inflammation, too. It does so through stabilizing blood pressure and fighting off radical elements.

- **Improved Skin Care**

Most of us are very self-conscious about how we look to the world. Bad skin, acne, and other skin ailments can be a real bother. Fasting has numerous benefits when it comes to improving your skin health, and it is said that fasting bestows a glow on your face. Experts claim that skin ailments develop as a result of terrible stomach environments and that there is a correlation between gut health and skin quality. Fasting promotes the development of gut flora. In this way, your gut health is improved, resulting in improved skin.

When you are on a fast and are taking water, you will eliminate toxins from your body. The condition of your skin improves because the skin cells are free of harmful substances. Many people who previously suffered from a bad skin condition and had tried almost every treatment with no success have admitted that fasting was the only thing that worked.

Another benefit of fasting is that it slows down the aging process. The water consumed during the fast goes to flush out toxins, consequently reducing the effects of old age on your skin. Fasting also promotes low blood sugar. Low blood sugar promotes optimized physiological processes and, as a result, toning down the effects of aging.

When you go on a fast, the body allocates energy to areas that might have previously been overlooked. So, your bad skin condition may be treated with the stored up energy, and considering that the energy produced from fat is more stable and resourceful; your skin health will improve.

- **Autophagy**

This is the process whereby the body rids itself of weakened and damaged cells. Autophagy is triggered by dry fasting. The body simply "eats" the weakened cells to provide water to the healthy cells. Eliminated cells are usually weak and damaged. And their absence creates room for new cells that are obviously going to be powerful.

Autophagy has been shown to have many benefits, and they include:

- **Slowing down aging effects**

  The formation of wrinkles and body deterioration are some of the effects of aging. However, thanks to autophagy, these effects can be reversed, since the body will destroy its old and weakened cells and replace them with new cells.

- **Reducing inflammation**

Inflammation is responsible for many diseases affecting us today, but thanks to autophagy, the cells that have been affected by inflammation are consumed, giving room for new cells.

- **Conserving energy**

Autophagy elevates the body into a state of energy conservation. In this way, your body can utilize resources in a most careful manner.

- **Fighting infections**

The destruction of old and weak body cells creates room for fresh and powerful body cells. In that vein, old and weakened white blood cells are destroyed, and then new powerful white blood cells are formed. These new white new blood cells fortify the immune system.

- **Improving motor skills**

Autophagy plays a critical role in improving the motor skills of an individual. This goes toward boosting the strength and agility of a person. Energy drawn from the weak and damaged cells is way more resourceful than the energy drawn from sugars.

Summary

There are numerous benefits attached to fasting. One of them is increased insulin sensitivity. When the insulin sensitivity goes up, insulin resistance drops, and the body is now able to use less insulin to convert sugars into energy. Another benefit of fasting is improved leptin sensitivity. The leptin hormone is known as the satiation hormone, and it is responsible for alerting you when you are full. An improved ghrelin level is another benefit of fasting. The ghrelin hormone is known as the hunger hormone. It induces hunger pangs so that you may feed. Fasting lengthens your existence. This is largely because of neuroregeneration of cells and flushing out toxins. Fasting improves brain function, strengthens your body and boosts agility, strengthens your immune system, optimizes your physiological functions, improves cardiovascular health, lowers blood pressure, reduces inflammation, improves your skin, and promotes autophagy. As researchers carry out new experiments, more benefits of fasting are being uncovered.

Chapter 4: Myths and Dangers of Fasting

Long-Held Myths and Misconceptions about Fasting

Fasting has gained widespread acceptance across the world. More people who are seeking to improve their health through alternative means are turning to fasting. As you might expect, the field has been marred with conspiracies, lies, half-truths, and outright ignorance. Some of the long-held myths and misconceptions about fasting include:

Fasting makes you overeat. This myth hinges on the idea that after observing a fast, an individual is bound to be so hungry that they will consume more food to compensate for the period they'd abstained from food.

The brain requires a steady supply of sugars. Some people say that the brain cannot operate normally in the absence of sugars. These people believe that the brain uses sugars alone to power its activities and any other source of energy would not be compatible. So when you fast, you'd be risking shutting down your brain functions.

Skipping breakfast will make you fat. Some people seem to treat breakfast as though it were an unexplained mystery of the Earth. They say breakfast is special. Anyone who misses breakfast cannot possibly have a healthy life. They say that if you skip breakfast, you will be under a heavy spell of cravings, and finally give in to unhealthy foods.

Fasting promotes eating disorders. Some people seem to think that fasting is the stepping stone for disorders like bulimia and anorexia. They complain that once you see the effects of fasting, you might want to "amplify" the effects which might make you susceptible to an eating disorder like anorexia.

Busting Myths Associated with Fasting

Fasting will make you overeat. This is partly true. However, it is important to note that most people fall into the temptation of overeating because of their lack of discipline and not necessarily because of unrealistic demands of fasting. If you're fasting the proper way, no temptation is big enough to lead you astray, and after all, the temptation exists to test whether you're really disciplined.

The brain requires a steady supply of sugars. This myth perpetuates the notion that we should consume carbohydrates every now and again to keep the brain in working condition. Also, this myth suggests that the brain can only use energy derived from sugars and not energy derived from fats. When you go on a fast, and your body uses up all the glycogen, your liver produces ketone bodies that are passed on to your brain to act as an energy source.

Skipping breakfast will make you fat. There is nothing special about breakfast. You can decide to skip breakfast and adhere to your schedule and be able to get desired results. It's true that skipping breakfast will cause you to be tempted by cravings, but you're not supposed to give in, and in that case, you become the problem. Skipping breakfast will not make you fat. What will make you fat is you pouring more calories into your body than you will spend.

Fasting promotes eating disorders. If you have a goal in mind, you are supposed to stay focused on that goal. The idea that an individual would plunge into the world of eating disorders simply because they want to amplify the results of fasting sounds like weakness on the part of the individual and not a fault of the practice itself.

Dangers of Fasting

Just as with most things in life, there's both a positive and negative side to fasting. Most of these problems are amplified in people who either fast in the wrong way or people who clearly shouldn't be fasting.

So let's explore some of the risks that are attached to fasting.

- **Dehydration**

Chances are, you will suffer dehydration while observing a fast, and drinking regular cups of water won't make the situation any better. Well, this is because most of your water intake comes from the foods that you consume daily. When dehydration kicks in, you are bound to experience nausea, headaches, constipation, and dizziness.

- **Orthostatic Hypotension**

This is common in people who drink water during their fasts. Orthostatic Hypotension causes your body to react unfavorably when you move around. For instance, when you stand on your feet and walk around, you might experience dizziness and feel as though you're at the verge of blowing up into smithereens. Other symptoms include temporary mental blindness, lightheadedness, and vision problems. These symptoms make it hard for you to function in activities that demand precision and focus, e.g., driving.

- **Worsened medical conditions**

People who fast while they are sick put themselves at risk of worsening their condition. The fast may amplify the symptoms of their diseases. People with the following ailments should first seek doctor's approval before getting into fasting: gout, type 2 diabetes, chronic kidney disease, eating disorders, and heartburn.

- **Increased stress**

The habit of skipping meals might lead to increased stress. The body might respond to hunger by increasing the hormone cortisol which is responsible for high-stress levels. And when you are in a stressed mental state, it becomes difficult to function in your day to day life.

Summary

Although fasting has a lot of benefits, there is a dark side to it too, but the negative effects can be minimized or eliminated altogether when a professional is involved. Dehydration is one of the negative effects. Besides providing nutrients to the body, food is also an important source of water. So when you fail to correct this gap by drinking a lot more water, your body will fall into a state of dehydration. Orthostatic hypotension is another danger. This illness makes you feel dizzy and lightheaded, and so it makes it difficult for you to function in an activity that demands your focus and stamina. Fasting may amplify the symptoms of your disease depending on your age and the stage of your disease. For instance, people who suffer from illnesses like gout, diabetes, eating disorders, and heartburn should first seek the doctor's approval before going on a fast. Moreover, fasting may lead to an increase in stress levels.

Chapter 5: Safety, Side Effects, and Warning

The Safest and Enlightened Way of Fasting

As the subject of fasting becomes popular, more people are stating their opinions on it, and as you might expect, some people are for it, and others are against it.

The best approach toward fasting is not set in stone, but it is rather determined by factors such as your age and health status.

Before you get into fasting, there are some critical balances you need to consider first. One of them is your experience. If you have never attempted a fast before, then it is a bad idea to go straight into a 48-hour fast, because you are likely to water down the effects. As a beginner, you must always start with lighter fasts and build your way up into extended fasts. You could begin by skipping one meal, then two meals, and finally the whole day.

Another important metric when it comes to determining the appropriate space between your eating windows is your health status. For instance, you cannot be a sufferer of late-stage malaria and yet go on a fast, because it might create a multiplying effect on your symptoms. People who are malnourished or have eating disorders might want to find other ways of improving their health apart from fasting.

An essential thing to note is that we are not all alike. My body's response to a fast is not going to be the exact response of yours. Knowing this, always listen to your body. Sometimes, a water-fast might trigger a throat infection and make your throat swollen. In such a situation, it would be prudent to suspend the fast and take care of your throat, as opposed to sticking to your guns.

Side Effects of Fasting

Fasting might upset the physiological functions of a body. This explains the side effects that crop up when you go on a fast. It is also important to note that most of these side effects subside as your body grows accustomed to the fast.

- **Cravings**

Top on the list is cravings. When you go on a fast, the immediate response by the body is to elevate the "hunger hormone" and so, you will start craving for sweet unhealthy foods. If you are not the disciplined type, this is a huge pitfall that could negate the effects of your fast.

- **Headaches**

Headaches, too, are a side effect of fasting. Most people who are new to fasting are bound to experience a headache. One of the explanations for headaches is that it is the brain's response to a shift from relying on carbohydrates to ketone bodies as the alternative energy source. Regular consumption of water might mitigate the headache or eliminate it altogether.

- **Low energy**

Another side effect is low energy. When you fast, the body might interpret it as starving, and its first response will be conserving energy. So, there will be less energy for physiological functions. In this way, you will start feeling less energetic than before.

- **Irritability**

Irritability is also a side effect. Studies show that people who are new to fasting are bound to have foul moods as their body increases stress hormones and hunger hormones. However, if they can persist, the irritability will eventually go away, and make room for a happy mood as the body switches to its fat stores for energy.

Types of People That Should Not Fast

The ideal person to go on a fast is a healthy person. People with certain medical conditions may still go on a fast, but it is always prudent to seek the guidance of a medical professional. We have previously stated that fasting strengthens the immune system. So is it contradicting to discourage fasting when one is sick? No! You may fast but preferably under the instruction and supervision of a medical professional. However, there are cases when it is inappropriate to fast.

Infants and children. Putting kids on a fast is just wrong. Their bodies are not fully developed yet to withstand periods of hunger. Fasting would do them more damage than good. For instance, it might mess with their metabolism and have a negative impact on their growth curve.

Hypoglycemics. People with hypoglycemia have extremely low levels of blood sugar. Their bodies need a constant stream of sugars to sustain normal functions lest severe illnesses take reign. For that reason, hypoglycemics should not fast.

Pregnant and nursing women. These women need a lot of energy because their young ones are dependent on them. So, pregnant women and nursing women are encouraged to keep their blood sugar steady.

The malnourished. People who are underweight and malnourished should stay away from fasting. To start with, their bodies don't have sufficient fat. So, when they go on a fast, their body will destroy its cells in search of nutrients. Over time, the results could be fatal.

People with heartburn. People who experience severe heartburn should not fast. This is because heartburn is a very distressing thing and there is no guarantee it will subside even when your body adapts to fasting. So, it is better to stay clear.

Impaired immune system. Fasting may have the ability to renew the strength and utility of your immune system. But when we are talking about an impaired immune system where most of the white blood cells are hanging on a thin blade, then fasting cannot be of help. Such a person would be better off sticking to a healthy diet.

Other classes of people that shouldn't fast include those recovering from surgeries, people with eating disorders, depressed souls, and people with extreme heart disease.

Summary

For purposes of safety, always ensure that your body is prepared to withstand the effects of fasting. You may prepare by evaluating your health status, experience, and developing a great sense of self-awareness. Fasting may have its numerous benefits, but there is also a negative side to it because fasting comes with unpleasant side effects. The good thing though is that most of these side effects tend to subside once the body grows accustomed to your fasting routine. One of the side effects of fasting is getting a headache. A headache is triggered by the brain's adjustment from relying on carbohydrates as an energy source and switching to ketone bodies. It may be mitigated through constant consumption of water. Another side effect is cravings. Your body makes you want to eat fast foods very badly. Fasting may also make you irritable, but it is for only a short time and then a happy mood sets in. Fasting also makes you feel less energetic, which can be uninspiring. These are some of the people that shouldn't fast: hypoglycemics, infants, children, pregnant women, nursing women, the malnourished, people with extreme ailments, and those recovering from surgeries.

PART 4.2

Types of Fasting and How to Fast

Chapter 6: Intermittent Fasting

What Is Intermittent Fasting?

Nowadays, intermittent fasting is one of the most talked about practices in health improvement domains. Basically, intermittent fasting is about creating a routine where you eat only after a set period of time. Intermittent fasting has been shown to have numerous benefits such as improving motor skills, developing willpower, and brain functions. Most people are turning to the practice to achieve their health goals—specifically, weight loss.

The most common way of performing an intermittent fast is by skipping meals. In the beginning, you may decide to skip one of the main meals, and when your body adapts to two meals a day, you may then elevate to just one meal per day. During the fast, you are not supposed to partake of any food, but it is okay to drink water and other low-calorie drinks like black coffee or black tea.

Intermittent fasting allows you to indulge in the foods of your choice, but there's emphasis on avoiding foods that are traditionally bad for your health. The main thing is to give your body time to process food between your eating windows.

Polls answered by people who have adopted this lifestyle indicate that most of them are happy with the results. Intermittent fasting is a very effective means of weight loss as it improves the metabolic rate of the body, as well as triggers cell autophagy. The good thing about intermittent fasting is that it allows you to partake of your favorite foods without making you feel guilty, which is a contrast to fad diets that insist on eating things like raw food and plant-based foods.

How to Practice Intermittent Fasting

There are a couple of ways to practice intermittent fasting. These are the three most popular ways:

- **The 16/8 method**

In this method, you are supposed to fast for 16 hours. Your eating window is restricted to eight hours every day. For instance, you might choose to only eat between twelve noon and eight in the evening.

- **Eat-Stop-Eat**

This fast involves irregular abstinence from food for a full 24 hours. You might decide to practice this once or twice every week. But when you fast, you must wait for 24 hours to pass before you indulge in the next meal. The eat-stop-eat method is very effective in not only weight loss but also in flushing out toxins from the body over the 24 hours you abstained from food.

- **The 5:2 Diet**

This type of intermittent fasting demands that you devote two days every week where you'll consume not more than 600 calories. Considering that the daily caloric requirement for the average person is 2000–2500, this type of fast will create a caloric deficit, and there's going to be weight loss as the body taps into its fat reservoirs for energy.

- **Alternate-Day Fasting**

This type of fasting requires that you skip one day and fast the next day. Depending on the intensity you want, you might choose to have a zero calorie intake or restrict your calorie intake to not more than 600. Alternate-day fasting is suitable for people who have experience with fasting and only want to escalate to amplify the benefits. A newbie should start with small fasts.

Pros and Cons of Intermittent Fasting

Intermittent fasting helps you save up on weekly food costs. That's a big advantage in these hard economic times. Food can be a very expensive affair especially if you eat out.

Intermittent fasting allows you to focus on your life goals. The energy that would have gone into looking for or preparing your next meal is used up to attain your important goals. Intermittent fasting has the potential to improve your emotional being and reduce anxiety—all of which make your life more stress-free.

Intermittent fasting is doable and safe. This means that it is free of complications and there's nothing to hold back anyone that wants to go into it. This is unlike other methods of weight loss like fad diets where some foods might be hard to access or expensive, or you dislike them.

Intermittent fasting improves the body's sensitivity to insulin, and by extension, it improves the metabolic rate of your body.

Moving on to the cons—the biggest disadvantage of intermittent fasting is the social dynamics. For instance, you might be out with friends when they decide to "pop in a joint" and then it's going to be strange to explain that you won't eat or maybe you'll defy your fasting routine and eat anyway, in which case you have cheated yourself.

Intermittent fasting doesn't seem to have a coherent and stable method. There are so many variations that dilute the philosophy of fasting. It almost feels like I can even come out with my style and popularize it. So, intermittent fasting lacks in originality.

Finding Your Ideal Intermittent Fasting Plan

The first and most important thing is to determine your health condition. If your body can permit you to indulge in intermittent fasting then, by all means, go ahead. If you are a beginner, you should start small, which means don't go from regular meals and start practicing 24-hour fasts. That's counterproductive. Make sure you have some experience before you fast for an extended period of time.

You'll find that what works for someone won't necessarily work for everybody else. So what's one supposed to do? Test, test, test. At one point you will find a variation of the intermittent fast that will fit perfectly into your life. It's all about finding what really works for you and then committing to the routine.

In my experience, I have found the 16:8 to be the best. This type of intermittent fast requires that you abstain from food for 16 hours and then indulge for 8 hours. For most followers of this routine, they like to have their eating window between 12:00 PM and 20:00 PM. The 16-hour fast will be inclusive of sleep, which makes it less severe.

This method is extremely efficient in weight loss, and most people have reported success. However, you must stick to the routine for a while before you can see any results. Don't do it for just one day and climb on the weighing machine only to find that there are no changes and then give up.

To improve the success of fasting intermittently, stick to a balanced diet during your eating windows, and don't take the fast as an excuse for indulging in unhealthy foods.

Step-By-Step Process of Fasting For a Week

The first step is to certify that you are in perfect condition. Get an appointment with your doctor and perform a whole health analysis to get a clean bill of health. Remember to always start with a small fast and gradually build up.

- **Day one**

When you wake up, forgo breakfast and opt for a glass of water or black coffee. Then go on about your work as you normally do. Around noon, your eating window opens. Now you are free to indulge in the food of your choice, but make sure that they are nutritious foods because unhealthy foods will water down your efforts. Your eating window should close at 20:00 PM, and from 20:01 pm to 12:00 pm the next day, don't consume anything else besides water.

- **Day two**

On day two, your body should have started to protest over the sudden calorie reduction, and so you'll be likely experiencing an irritable mood, lightheadedness, and a small headache. When you wake up, no matter how strong the urge to eat might be, just push it back, and the only thing you should consume is water or black coffee. At noon, your eating window opens, and you're free to eat until 8 pm.

- **Day three**

When you wake up, take a glass of water or black coffee. Chances are that your body has started to adjust to the reduced daily caloric intake. It has switched to burning fats. At twelve noon, when your eating window opens, consume less food than you did yesterday and the day before, so that the body has even lesser calories to work with. The body should adapt to this pretty swiftly.

- **Day four**

In the morning, take a glass of water or black coffee and go about your business. When your eating window opens, eat as much food as you ate yesterday, but in the evening, resist the urge to drink anything.

- **Day five**

When you wake up, take a glass of water or black coffee. During your eating window, eat less food than you did previously. At night, resist the urge to drink water.

- **Day six**

When you wake up, resist the urge to drink water or even coffee. In your eating window, choose not to eat at all, and at night give in to the temptation and drink water or black coffee.

- **Day seven**

When you wake up, take a glass of water or black coffee. In your eating window, resume eating, but only take a small portion, and just before you close the eating window, eat again, except it should be a slightly larger meal than previously. Before you sleep, take another glass of water or black coffee. Fast till your next eating window, and then you may resume your normal eating habits. At this point, you will have lost weight and experienced a host of other benefits attached to intermittent fasting.

Summary

Intermittent fasting features a cycle of fasting interrupted by an eating window. Some of the methods of intermittent fasting include the 16:8, eat-stop-eat, 5:2, and alternate-day fasting. The best approach to intermittent fasting is context-based in the sense that only you can know what works for you. The most popular form of intermittent fasting is the 16:8. In this method, you fast for 16 hours and then an eating window of 8 hours. The biggest advantage of intermittent fasting is that it announces relief to your pocket. The "food budget" goes into other uses. The amount of time that it takes to prepare meals is a real hassle, but intermittent fasting frees up your time so you can be more productive. The entry barrier is nonexistent too. This means anyone can practice intermittent fasting because there are no barriers or things to buy—a stark contrast to other weight loss methods like fad diets that may be both inconveniencing and expensive.

Chapter 7: Longer Periods of Fasting

What is Fasting for Longer Periods?

Fasting for longer periods is reserved for people who have a bit of experience with fasting. A newbie shouldn't get into it.

It is basically desisting from food for not less than 24 hours, but not more than, say, 48 hours. You may increase the success of the fast by making it a dry fast. In a dry fast, you won't have the luxury of drinking water or any other low-calorie drink like black coffee.

Fasting for longer periods requires that you prepare emotionally, mentally, and physically. The buildup to your fast is an especially important part. Your food consumption should be minimal.

Fasting for a longer period helps you achieve much more results because the body will be subjected to an increased level of strain.

However, you must take care to know when to stop. In some instances, the body might rebel by either catching an infection or shutting down critical functions, and in such times it is prudent to call off the fast.

During longer fasts, you should abstain from strenuous exercises, because the body will be in a state of energy conservation, and the available energy is purposed for physiological functions.

With the wrong approach, long fasts might become disastrous. That's why it is always important to seek clearance from your doctor first before you go into the fast. And to flush out toxins, ensure you have a steady intake of water.

It is estimated that weight loss in longer fasts averages around one to two pounds every day.

How to Fast for Longer Periods

The main reason that people go into longer fasts is to obviously lose weight. But you might want to fast to reach other purposes such as flushing toxins from your body or heightening your mental capabilities. Also, a longer fast is recommended if you are going into a surgery.

The response to a fast is different for everyone. If it is your first time, please take great care by getting medical clearance.

As your fast approaches, you might want to minimize your food consumption to get used to managing hunger.

Next, you should clear away items that might ruin your focus or tempt you to backslide. You might want to give your kitchen a total makeover by, for instance, clearing away the bad food. It is much easier to manage cravings when they are out of sight than when they are within easy reach.

Always start small. Before you deprive yourself food for over 24 hours, you should first get a taste of what food deprivation for 8 hours feels like, and if you can handle that, then you're ready to step up your game. While you fast, you should be very aware of the ranges of effects that your body experiences. You might feel dizzy, lightheaded, sleepy, or distressed, and these are okay reactions. Things that are not okay are infections and prolonged aches of body parts. If your body responds to fasting unfavorably, you should stop the fast.

Pros and Cons of Fasting for Longer Periods

If you have always been motivated to clear away the stubborn fat in your body, but have never found an efficient method, then the answer is to fast for a longer period.

When you go on a longer fast, the body uses up all glycogen in the first 24 hours, and then it switches to burning fats. A longer fast guarantees quick weight loss.

A longer fast saves you money. Food is an expensive affair, especially if you eat out. With a longer fast, it means you are staying away from food, and are thus saving on food costs.

Besides the benefit of optimizing your health, a longer fast will strengthen both your willpower and mental sharpness, which are two necessary factors in attaining success.

Fasting for a longer period helps you appreciate the taste of food. By the time you're done fasting, you'll want to indulge your appetite, and food will suddenly taste so sweet. The scarcity factor elevates the value of food.

A longer fast has cons, too. One of the biggest cons is the strain that it puts on your body. When your body goes from relying on glycogen into fats as a source of energy, nasty side effects are bound to come up—for instance, headaches, nausea, and lightheadedness.

Another con is that fasting for a longer period might open you up to disease. As much as fasting renews your immune system, your body still needs robust energy to function optimally. Fasting puts your body into a state of conserving energy which makes it easy for disease to attack.

Step-By-Step Process of Fasting for Longer Periods

When you decide to go on a fast for a longer period, you must realize that you are signing up for a real challenge. The body's immediate response to a fast is raising the hunger hormone to alert you to look for food. Now, fighting off that urge takes a lot of willpower. In some regard, it's why fasting might be considered a test of discipline because not so many people can withstand it.

So here's the step-by-step process of going on a fast for longer periods:

Preparation

The first major thing is to ensure that your body is in a condition that will allow you to fast, without any complications. In other words, consult your doctor for a checkup.

Reduce your food intake in the days leading up to your fast so that your body can get accustomed to staying without food. Once your body is familiar with the feeling of food deprivation, you are ready to move forward.

In the morning of your fast, drink lots of water. It is critical for flushing out toxins and reducing stomach acidity when your stomach secretes acids in anticipation of food. Your water intake should be regular and spread out through the day.

Rather than lying down and wearing a look of self-pity, just go on about your work as you normally would, provided it is not a very focus-oriented job like performing surgeries.

You should stay the whole day without food and then go to bed. On the following morning, your hunger pangs will be even more amplified, at which point you are to mitigate the hunger with a drink of water and then maintain the fast for another 24 hours. 48 hours are enough for a longer fast, and the weight loss should be dramatic. After the fast, don't immediately go back to eating heavy amounts of food, but rather ease your way into a lighter diet.

Chapter 8: Extended Fasting

How to Fast for Extended Periods

Fasting for an extended period is an extreme form of fasting that demands you abstain from food from anywhere between three days to seven days. If you can deny yourself food for more than three days, you should be proud of yourself, because not so many people have that kind of determination.

Fasting for an extended period of time amplifies the results of a longer fast. When you go for an extended period of time without food, you will allow yourself to experience a range of different feelings. At the initial stage there is distress, and towards the end your feelings become tranquil.

Considering that this is an especially long fast, you are supposed to take a very keen listen to the response by your body. If your body sends out the message that it is under massive strain, now it's time to stop the fast. Cases where it's appropriate to stop include developing stomach ulcers, throat infection, and loss of consciousness.

You should eat lighter meals as you approach the start of your fast. During the fast, your water intake should be regular. When you complete the fast, the transition to your normal eating life should be slow and gradual, starting with lighter meals.

Fasting for an extended period has the biggest potential of going wrong. The prolonged food deprivation in itself may do more good than harm. There is also the possibility of slightly altering your body's physiological functions. Still, the benefits of an extended fast outweigh the negatives.

Pros and Cons of Fasting for Extended Periods

The biggest advantage of fasting for an extended period of time is the discipline it instills in you. When you go for a prolonged period without eating food, your body will respond by increasing hunger pangs. It takes extreme willpower to keep going. This experience can help you build your self-control and discipline in real life.

An extended fast is very effective in banishing stubborn fat. Most people who are obese will tell you that they are trying to lose weight, but the fat is stubborn. Guess what, their methods are ineffective. However, if they had the will and courage to go on an extended fast, then they'd experience a rapid weight loss and reach their desired weight.

Extended fasting promotes a high rate of cell replenishing. When the body goes for days without food, it turns in on itself and begins to digest its cells—the weak and damaged cells—to provide nutrition for the healthy cells. The elimination of weak and damaged cells creates room for new and healthy ones.

The biggest disadvantage for an extended period of fasting is the risk of complications that you put your body into. Some complications might be instant whereas others may develop long after the fast. The biggest risk is catching an infection. If you're unlucky enough that you catch some disease in your fast, your immune system will be overwhelmed.

Another huge miss about extended fasting is the disconnect it encourages in your normal life. When you are fasting, you won't be able to share a meal with your friends or family, and that can be a big inconvenience. It can make people "talk."

Step-By-Step Process of Fasting for Extended Periods

When you get clearance from a medical professional, you should start by preparing for the extended fast. Ideally, if you are getting into an extended fast, you should have experience with either intermittent fasting, longer fasting or both. The more your body is familiar with food deprivation, the better the outcome.

On the start of your extended fast, you should consume only water or black coffee, and throughout the rest of the day, observe regular water consumption. It will aid in flushing out toxins and other harmful elements from your body.

During the fast, you should keep your normal work schedule, as opposed to being inactive, because inactivity will worsen your hunger pangs. The standard response to hunger pangs should be water consumption.

On the second day, first thing in the morning is to consume more water. This water is very critical in flushing out toxins and keeping your body cells hydrated as well as regulating autophagy. However, if you want to increase the success rate of the fast, you might consider eliminating water. One of the side effects of this type of fast is a dry mouth. A dry mouth has the potential of being very distressing. For purposes of safety, always hydrate yourself.

On the third day, wake up and consume water or black coffee. At this point, your body is subsisting on its fat reserves, and the weight loss is evident. Your body has potentially minimized hunger pangs to manageable levels. Keep yourself busy. Otherwise, inactivity will provoke hunger.

From the fourth day up until the seventh, keep the same routine. When you come to the end of your fast, realize that your body will be in starvation mode, so don't immediately consume large amounts of food. Instead, ease your way back into a normal eating schedule.

Chapter 9: The Eating Window

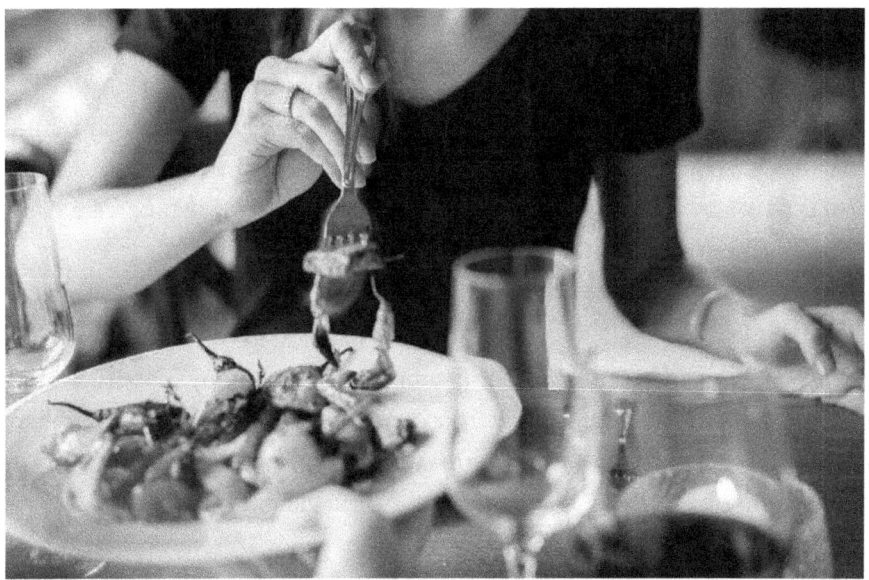

What is the Eating Window?

The eating window is the period of time that you are allowed to indulge in foods and one that precedes a period of fasting. The eating window comes around on a cycle, and you should adhere to it by only eating when the window opens and abstaining from food the rest of the time.

The hours are not set in stone. You are free to choose your eating window in a way that works for you. Most people who practice intermittent fasting seem to adhere to an eight-hour eating window followed by a sixteen-hour fast. Commonly, the eight-hour window opens at around 12:00 PM and goes all the way to 20:00 PM. During this time, you may indulge in your favorite foods. However, past 20:00 PM, you are supposed to observe the fast.

The 16:8 method of intermittent fasting appeals to many people because the 16 hours of fasting are inclusive of the bed-time. If you are not into waiting for sixteen hours before you partake of food, you may lessen the hours, so that you will have frequent eating windows between your fasts.

It is generally more fruitful to have a small eating window followed by a long period of fast.

It's also important to choose an eating window that optimizes your health. For instance, eating during the day is of much benefit than eating at night. This is because the body puts more calories to use during the day as opposed to while you are asleep. Also, adhere to a good diet, or else your gains will be neutralized by a bad diet.

What to Eat

The reason why intermittent fasting appeals to so many people is the nonexistent dietary rules common in alternative weight loss methods like fad diets. In intermittent fasting, you are free to eat the foods of your choice, and the main thing is to restrict your caloric intake.

You are free to consume the foods that delight you, but be careful not to fall in the pit of overcompensation. You are at risk of misleading yourself into consuming unhealthy foods during your eating window under the delusion that fasting will take care of it. Truth is, some of the fast foods we indulge are so calorie-laden that it would take a prolonged fast (not intermittent) to eliminate their fat from our bodies.

Limit your intake of red meat. As much as intermittent fasting is lenient when it comes to diet, it is widely known that red meat causes more harm than good. So, you might want to limit its intake or eliminate it altogether.

Fruits are a source of essential nutrients for the body. Always make sure to include fruits like bananas, avocados, and apples into your meals. Fruits help reduce inflammation and are critical in optimizing the physiological functions of the body.

Vegetables should be in your meals. People who claim that vegetables taste bad are just unimaginative cooks. Vegetables do taste good. And some of the health benefits of vegetable include strengthening your bones, stabilizing your blood sugar, boosting your brain health, and improving your digestive system.

Developing Discipline

It takes a lot of discipline to persevere through a fast. Think about it. The average person is accustomed to eating something every now and then. They cannot afford to hold back for even a couple more hours when lunch is due. The eating cycle never ends. And so a person who can decide to abstain from food and stick to their decision is a special kind of person—he/she is disciplined.

The biggest challenge when it comes to fasting for an extended period is to overcome the hunger pangs over the first few days. Your body floods you with the hunger hormone, pushing you to look for food. However, if you persevere through the first few days, your body will adjust to the food deprivation and switch to your stored fats as the alternative source of energy.

One of the things you must do to boost your self-control is to prepare your mind. When you have an idea of what to expect, the hunger will be more tolerable as opposed to if you're ignorant. Another thing to take into consideration is the weather. You don't want to fast during a cold season because fasting lowers your body temperature, and so you'll be hard-hit.

Another way of boosting your discipline is joining hands with people of the same goal. In this way, you can keep each other in check. When you are on a team or have a friend who practices fasting too, it will be easy to stick to your plan, as everybody will offer psycho-social support to everybody else. Sometimes, the difference between throwing in the towel and sticking to your guns is a kind word of encouragement.

Summary

The eating window is the period of time that you are allowed to indulge in foods and one that precedes a period of fasting. The eating window comes around on a cycle, and you should adhere to it by only eating when the window opens and abstaining from food the rest of the time.

Intermittent fasting doesn't restrict the consumption of certain foods as is common for other weight loss methods such as fad diets. To boost the effectiveness of your fast, your diet should be balanced, which means it should include foods rich in minerals and vitamins. There also should be fruits and vegetables. Discipline is very important when it comes to fasting. It's what keeps you going when your body protests hunger. The most important step toward developing discipline is to first prepare mentally for the fast. Another way of developing discipline is by having a strong support system.

PART 4.3

Targeted Fasting for Your Body Type

Chapter 10: Fasting For Weight Loss

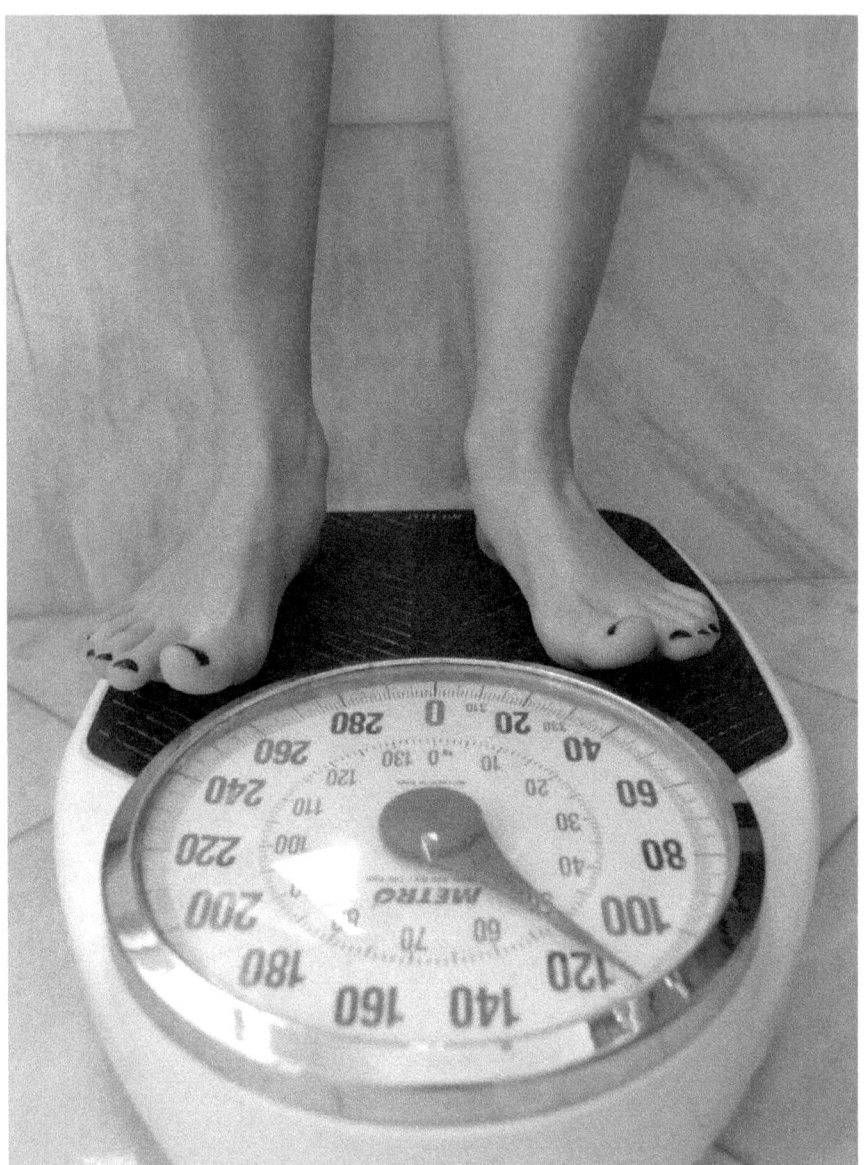

Why You'll Lose Weight through Fasting

Some of the methods of losing weight include fad diets, exercising, and supplements. However, these methods are not very effective, and in most cases, they cannot solve obesity on their own.

Fasting is easily the best method of not only reducing weight but also eliminating the stubborn lower-stomach fat. But why is it so?

First off, fasting optimizes the biological functions of your body. Fasting allows you to ease the load on your digestive system. The spare energy goes toward optimizing your physiological functions. For instance, improved digestion streamlines your bowel movement too. This efficacy in the physiological functions creates a compounding effect that leads to the shedding of dead weight, thus reducing an individual's weight and actually stabilizing it.

Another way in which fasting promotes weight loss is through cell autophagy. A dry fast is particularly what triggers cell autophagy. When the body uses up all its water, it now starts digesting the weak and damaged cells to provide water for the body cells that are in a much better state. Autophagy helps in eliminating dead and weak cells thereby making a person lighter.

Fasting plays a critical role in improving the metabolic health of an individual. With improved metabolism, the body can crunch more calories, and thus the individual's weight goes down.

Fasting improves insulin sensitivity. This helps the body to convert more sugars into energy. The body uses more calories, and as a result, there's a loss of weight.

In most obese people, the communication between their brain and ghrelin cells is warped, which makes them experience hunger all the time, even when they are full. Fasting helps remedy this problem, and obese people start receiving accurate signals when they are hungry.

Step-By-Step Process of Losing Weight through Fasting

- **Checkup**

First off, make sure that your body is in a condition that allows you to fast. Some of the people who are discouraged from the practice include pregnant women, nursing women, infants, sufferers of late-stage terminal illnesses, and those who are recovering from surgery.

- **Water**

Your body will respond to food deprivation by secreting acids and enzymes, and for that reason, always start your fast with consuming water. Regular water consumption will flush out the toxins and will also ease you from stomach pain.

- **Eating window**

Desist from food for at least 16 hours and then take a meal of your choice. The ideal eating window should be around eight hours. During this eight hour break, you are free to indulge. However, you must take care not to consume unhealthy foods. They will just neutralize your fasting efforts. Also, mind the portions. Simply because you have eight hours to feed doesn't mean you should fill up that period with food only.

- **Exercise**

Taking aerobic exercises, in particular, will have a dramatic effect on your weight loss. Aerobic exercises act like a calorie furnace. Also, exercises will increase the toxins in your body, and for that reason, keep yourself hydrated.

- **Breaking the fast**

At the end of your fast, never go right back into "heavy eating," but rather ease your way back by first consuming lighter foods. It'd be prudent of you to make fasting a part of your lifestyle. The key thing is to go with works for you. Most people seem to prefer intermittent fasting because it can fit in most people's lives. Prolonged fasting should be done sparingly as it carries the risk of developing complications.

Summary

Fasting has a positive impact on the rate of metabolism. When the metabolism rate is high, the energy output of the body goes up, and thus more calories are used up. This creates a caloric deficit and subsequent weight loss. Fasting promotes cell autophagy. Autophagy is the process where weak and damaged body cells are digested by the body. The elimination of weak body cells helps in weight reduction. High insulin resistance makes it hard for the body cells to absorb the sugars in the blood. But fasting reduces insulin resistance so that the body will use less insulin to convert sugars into energy. Before you go on a fast, you should get medical clearance. Some of the people who shouldn't get into a fast include the terminally ill, pregnant women, nursing women, and people who are recovering from surgery. It is important to take water throughout the fast to flush out toxins and mitigate the effect of stomach acids.

Chapter 11: Fasting for Type 2 Diabetes

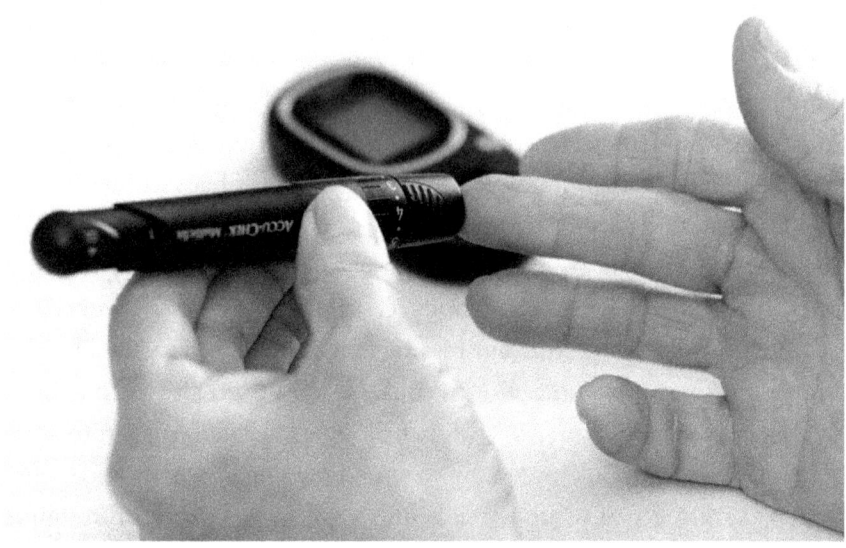

What is Type 2 Diabetes?

Type 2 diabetes is a disease that damages the ability of the pancreas to produce sufficient insulin. Insulin is the hormone produced by the pancreas, and its main function is to regulate the conversion of glucose into energy. The body cells of people who have type 2 diabetes are insensitive to insulin, and as such, they experience difficulty in converting sugars into energy. This condition is known as insulin resistance. It is characterized by the production of higher amounts of insulin, but the body cannot absorb it.

As to the origin of type 2 diabetes, scientists have established that it is genetic. The disease is handed down to progeny. Another leading cause of type 2 diabetes is obesity. Overweight people are much more likely to develop insulin resistance. There's a link between childhood obesity and development of type 2 diabetes in adulthood.

Another contributing factor is a metabolic syndrome. High insulin resistance is a result of increased blood pressure and cholesterol.

Excessive sugars produced by the liver may also be a trigger.

The symptoms of type 2 diabetes cover a wide range. They include thirst, frequent peeing, hazy vision, irritability, tiredness, and yeast infections.

The risk of developing type 2 diabetes can be greatly minimized by taking the following actions:

Losing weight. Weight loss improves insulin sensitivity, and thus the buildup of insulin in the blood is eliminated. Also, there's more conversion of sugars into energy.

Balanced diet. You should consume foods that are sources of minerals and vitamins. Increase your intake of fruits and vegetables. Minimize your consumption of sugars and red meat.

The Role of Insulin in the Body

The insulin hormone is produced by the pancreas. Its key role is to regulate blood sugar. Increased insulin resistance might lead to type 2 diabetes. Insulin plays the critical role of facilitating absorption of sugars into body cells. In this way, insulin helps to reduce the blood sugar level. Another important role of insulin is to modify the activity of enzymes. The enzymes are secreted by the body when there's food in the stomach. Insulin regulates the activity of enzymes.

Insulin helps the body recover quickly. When your body is recovering from an injury or illness, insulin plays a critical role in speeding up the healing process by transporting amino acids to cells.

Insulin promotes gut flora and thus improves gut health. This improves bowel movement. Insulin also improves the excretion of harmful substances like sodium.

Insulin promotes brain health. It improves brain clarity by providing the essential nutrients to the brain.

Insulin plays a key role in determining the metabolism rate of the body. In instances of high insulin sensitivity, the blood glucose is easily absorbed into the cells, making for a high metabolic rate. But in instances of low insulin sensitivity, the process of converting sugars into energy becomes hard, and, consequently, there is a low metabolic rate.

Insulin is very important in the optimal functioning of your body. Some of the factors that improve the production of the insulin hormone are having a balanced diet, improving your brain health, having quality sleep, exercising, and staying in a pollution-free environment.

How Diabetes Affects both Production and Usage of Insulin

Diabetes is a major lifestyle disease all over the world. A person who has diabetes either cannot produce sufficient insulin, or their body cells are insensitive to insulin. Diabetes is broadly classified into two types: type 1 and type 2.

People who suffer from type 1 diabetes produce little to no insulin. This slows down the rate of conversion of sugars into energy. A low level of insulin is mainly a result of the immune system attacking the pancreas and curtailing its ability to produce sufficient insulin. Also, low insulin levels might be a result of weakened and damaged body cells. Type 1 diabetes commonly affects young people. One of the corrective measures is to administer insulin through injections.

Symptoms of type 1 diabetes include dehydration, constant urge to urinate, hunger (even after eating), unexplained weight loss, blurry vision, exhaustion, and bad moods.

Type 2 diabetes is the most common form of diabetes. People who suffer from type 2 diabetes have a high insulin resistance. Their body cells are averse to insulin. Types 2 diabetes is treated by increasing insulin sensitivity.

Symptoms of type 2 diabetes include tiredness, never-ending thirst, constant urge to pee, irritability, weak immune, and shivering.

The pancreas is the organ that produces insulin. When we consume food, blood sugar rises. The pancreas releases insulin to facilitate the conversion of sugars into energy. But someone who suffers from diabetes either lacks sufficient insulin or their body cannot use the released insulin. This results in increased blood sugar levels. This scenario presents risks such as the development of heart disease and stroke.

How Blood Sugar Responds To Fasting

A carbohydrate metabolism test is crucial in determining how blood sugar responds to fasting. The test is conducted on diabetics. During a fast, the levels of plasma glucose go up. People with diabetes either cannot produce sufficient insulin, or their bodies are resistant to insulin. Non-diabetics, though, produce insulin that brings down the levels of glucose through absorption.

Diet greatly affects the blood sugar rate-of-increase. For instance, a big serving of food will trigger a high level of blood sugar, and sugar-laden foods like cake, bread, and fries will also increase the blood sugar level.

People with type 1 diabetes lack sufficient insulin because their immune system attacks the pancreas, while people with type 2 diabetes are insensitive to insulin. So in both cases, there is a high level of blood sugar.

The levels of blood glucose during fasting give us insight into how the cells respond to blood sugar. A high level of blood glucose is indicative of the body's ability to lower blood glucose, and the conclusion might be either high insulin resistance or insufficient insulin production. Prolonged fasting has the effect of minimizing blood glucose levels. The sugars in the blood get used up, albeit slowly.

There are two methods of testing the level of blood sugar: the traditional blood sugar test, and the glycosylated hemoglobin (HbAlc). The glycosylated hemoglobin test is for checking how blood glucose has been changing. The traditional method of checking blood sugar involves daily tests which may be conducted by the affected person.

Developing Your Fasting Regimen

There are some fasting regimens. All of them have their pros and cons. They are only as good as the person trying to follow them. During fasts, it is recommended to take water to flush out toxins and also to mitigate hunger. However, if you want to improve the success rate of your fast, you might consider dry fasts, where you don't consume any fluid.

You may perform a fast for as short a time as a couple of hours or as long as a full week (and maybe even more, depending on your stamina). However, if your goal is to lose weight, then shorter fasts are more effective. For instance, intermittent fasting is many times more fruitful than prolonged fasting, but ultimately, you get to choose what you feel will work for you.

Short fasts allow you to go through a cycle of fasting and eating windows. You start by creating a plan in which you detail your period of fasting and when your eating window opens. During the eating window, it is advisable to consume unprocessed foods and avoid sugar-laden foods. This will boost your insulin sensitivity.

Long fasts have their benefits too, but on the whole, they are much less rewarding than short fasts. The strain associated with long fasts make you susceptible to infections and might, in the worst case scenario, rewire your physiological functions.

Things to Incorporate to Make Fasting Safe for Diabetics

When a diabetic goes on a fast, their body secretes the glucagon hormone, which leads to a spike in the blood sugar level. Thus, a diabetic should start by informing themselves properly before they deprive themselves of food.

The first thing is to determine whether they are fit to fast. A diabetic person should seek medical clearance before they attempt fasting. A person with advanced diabetes will have a low blood sugar level. If they go on a fast, they risk falling into a coma. A medical professional offers the best counsel as to how to conduct the fast and for how long.

For type 1 diabetics, it is important to have a test kit to observe the fluctuation of blood sugar throughout the fast. This helps in tweaking the fast or deciding whether to call it off.

Another safety measure is to have a confidant know of their fasting. The psycho-social support offered by a confidant would keep them going. The confidant should be someone in their close proximity that can monitor their progress.

Diabetics should indulge in a balanced diet during their eating window. A balanced diet comprises of foods rich in minerals and vitamins. One common thing that fasting induces is cravings. Fast foods, for instance, are sugar-laden and they have no real nutritional value. Indulging in fast foods during eating windows only negates the effectiveness of the fast.

A diabetic should know when to quit and how to quit. If there is a massive fluctuation of blood glucose, or if a complication develops, then that's a hint to quit. Towards the end of the fast, a diabetic should consume light meals first, and then transition back to their normal eating patterns.

Role of Supplements

A supplement is a substance that enhances the food that a person eats. The common types of ingredients in supplements include vitamins, minerals, botanicals, amino acids, enzymes, organ tissues, and glandulars. The supplements are critical in optimizing nutritional value of food. The water-soluble ingredients of supplements are metabolized and eliminated from the body same day, while fat-soluble elements may be stored in the body for several days or even weeks. Supplements may be taken on either a daily basis or alternately—depending on the elements they provide to the body. One should always seek the guidance of a medical professional about the number of supplements to consume.

Supplements are not as critical during short fasts as they are in prolonged fasts. The body is a store of many nutritional elements, and fasting induces the body to tap into its reservoirs, but it is still important to take supplements to discourage nutrition deficiency. Fat-soluble vitamins need to be taken alongside fats to make for easy absorption. They include vitamin A, vitamin D, vitamin E, and vitamin K. They are kept in body cells too. Water-soluble vitamins are eliminated on the same day, especially if your body is well hydrated. Water-soluble vitamins include B3, B2, B1, and acids. If you have a poor diet, water-soluble vitamins are stable sources of nutrition.

The primary function of supplements is to improve the nutritional value of a person's diet by supplying vital elements that are not easily accessible. Taking supplements while on a fast helps mitigate the side effects of fasting such as headaches and cramps.

Types of Supplements that Stabilize Electrolytes

Sodium. The intake of Sodium is dependent upon your level of physical activity. Generally, if you engage in tougher physical exercises, you should take a high dose. Sodium is vital in eliminating cramps and various pains in the body.

Potassium. This supplement is vital for the optimal functioning of the heart. Potassium deficiency is normally accompanied by problems such as increased heartbeat and blood pressure. Potassium also helps in the flow of blood. A person with potassium deficiency is bound to experience exhaustion and constant lethargic feeling.

Magnesium. People who are lacking in this vital nutrient experience a range of problems like low energy, anxiety, insomnia, indigestion, muscle aches, poor heart health, and migraines. Magnesium supplements help your body absorb magnesium at a higher rate. Magnesium should be taken alongside food as opposed to plainly for maximum health benefit.

Zinc. This supplement is very crucial in improving the health of an individual. It regulates appetite, improves taste, promotes weight loss, minimizes hair loss, mitigates digestive problems, and cures chronic fatigue. Additionally, zinc improves nerve health and boosts testosterone. Zinc, too, should be consumed alongside other meals for maximum health benefits.

Calcium. This supplement helps in strengthening the musculoskeletal frame of an individual, heart health, and reduces the risk of developing ailments like cancer and diabetes. Calcium and magnesium should be taken at separate times to avoid stunted absorption rates.

Iodine. Iodine is crucial in improving thyroid health. The thyroid gland secretes hormones that play a vital role in the basal metabolic rate.

How to Keep Insulin Levels Low

This hormone produced by the pancreas facilitates the absorption of sugars into body cells. The insulin levels should be stable for optimum metabolism to take place. High levels of insulin might lead to serious complications like high blood pressure. Someone with a high blood glucose level needs to lower their blood sugar level, else they may suffer serious health complications. Here are some of the ways to keep insulin levels low.

Diet. Your diet will have a direct impact on your blood sugar levels. Sugary, fat-laden foods will raise your blood glucose through the roof. On the other hand, a low-carb diet will help keep your blood glucose levels down.

Portion. There is a direct correlation between the portion of your food and your blood sugar levels. A giant portion of your favorite dish will lead to a surge in blood glucose. On the other hand, a small portion will keep your blood sugar stable. Bearing this in mind, you should aim to take small portions of food, as they minimize the fluctuation of blood glucose levels.

Exercise regularly. You can bring the high blood sugar levels down through exercise. When you exercise, your body powers your activities with the glucose in your blood. So exercises—and in particular, aerobics—can lead to low blood glucose levels.

Drink water constantly. Staying hydrated is also important in keeping the blood sugar level down. Water will flush out toxins and help streamline your metabolism.

Avoid alcohol. Alcohol not only lowers your inhibitions and makes you indulge in unhealthy foods like fries and roast meat, but it is also calorie-packed. If you aim to minimize your blood sugar, restrict your alcohol intake or drop it altogether.

What Causes Insulin Resistance?

Insulin is produced by the pancreas, and its work is to facilitate absorption of glucose into body cells. Insulin resistance is a condition where body cells are insensitive to insulin. For that reason, the rate of conversion of sugars into energy is affected. What are some of the causes of this condition?

Obesity. Most obese people have a ton of toxic elements stashed in their body. The combination of high blood sugar levels and toxic elements promote cellular inflammation. These cells naturally become insulin resistant.

Inactivity. Insulin resistance is common in people who hardly ever move their limbs. They don't perform any physical activity, so their energy requirement (output) is minimal. This creates some sort of "cell apathy" and promotes insulin resistance.

Sleep apnea. This is a sleep disorder characterized by faulty breathing. People who suffer from sleep apnea snore loudly and also feel tired after a night's sleep. Studies have shown a link between sleep apnea and development of insulin resistance in body cells.

High blood pressure. High blood pressure or hypertension is a degenerative medical issue where the blood pressure in blood vessels is more than 140/90 mmHg. Hypertension makes the heart's task of pumping out blood more difficult and may contribute to complications such as atherosclerosis, stroke, and kidney disease. Studies have shown a correlation between people with high blood pressure and the development of insulin resistance.

Smoking. The habit of smoking can give you many health complications. One of them is the risk of cancer development. Additionally, smoking seems to promote insulin resistance.

How Insulin Resistance Affects the Body

Insulin resistance makes it hard for the body cells to absorb sugars, which leads to high blood glucose levels. Some of the causes of insulin resistance include obesity, poor diet, sleep disorders, and sedentary lifestyle.

The American Diabetes Association (ADA) has stated that there is a 70% chance for people with insulin resistance to develop type 2 diabetes if they don't change their habits.

Insulin resistance may trigger the development of acanthosis nigricans, a skin condition in which dark spots cover parts of the body, especially the neck region.

Insulin resistance enhances weight gain, because it slows down base metabolism, causing a surge of blood sugar levels. Insulin carries off the excess blood sugar into fat stores, and thus, the person gains weight.

Insulin resistance promotes high blood pressure. The elevated blood glucose levels cause the heart to have to struggle with pumping more blood, causing high blood pressure.

Insulin resistance causes constant thirst and hunger pangs. Insulin resistance promotes the miscommunication between brain receptors and body cells. Thus, the brain activates the hunger hormone and makes the person eternally hungry. If not corrected, this leads to overeating and eventually chronic obesity.

Insulin resistance weakens the body. Insulin resistance leads to low energy output. And for that reason, the body doesn't have a lot of energy to use up, which makes the person feel (and look) weak.

Insulin resistance makes you urinate frequently; the condition affects the efficiency of physiological functions, and one of the results is a constant need to urinate.

Insulin resistance makes the body more susceptible to attack by diseases.

The Role of Amylin

Amylin is a protein hormone. It is produced by the pancreas alongside insulin. Amylin helps in glycemic control by promoting the slow emptying of the gastric and giving feelings of satisfaction. Amylin discourages the upsurge of blood glucose levels.

Amylin is part of the endocrine system, and it plays a critical role in glycemic control. The hormone is secreted by the pancreas, and its main function is to slow down the rate of appearance of nutritional elements in the plasma. It complements insulin.

Amylin and Insulin are secreted in a ratio of 1:100. Amylin delays gastric emptying and decreases the concentration of glucose in the plasma, whereas insulin facilitates absorption of sugars into cells. Diabetic people lack this hormone.

The amylin hormone can coalesce and create amyloid fibers, which may help in destroying diabetes. Amylin is secreted when there is the stimulus of nutrition in the blood. Unlike insulin, it is not purged in the liver but by renal metabolism.

Recent studies have shown the effect of amylin on the metabolism of glucose. In rats, amylin promoted insulin resistance.

Amylin slows down the food movement through the gut. As the food stays longer in the stomach, the rate of conversion of these foods to sugars will be slower.

Amylin also prevents the secretion of glucagon. Glucagon causes a surge in blood sugar level. Amylin prevents the inappropriate secretion of glucagon, which might cause a post-meal spike in blood sugar.

Amylin enhances the feeling of satiety. By reducing appetite, amylin ensures low blood glucose levels.

How Amylin Deficiency Affects Your Body

Amylin regulates the concentration of glucose in the blood by preventing the secretion of glucagon and slowing down the movement of food along the gut. People who suffer from diabetes have an amylin deficiency that causes excessive amounts of glucose to flow into the blood.

Increased insulin. A deficiency in amylin causes an extreme surge in blood glucose levels. To mitigate this spike, the pancreas secretes more insulin to help in the absorption of sugars into body cells. Increased levels of insulin in the blood might lead to complications.

Insulin resistance. Amylin deficiency eventually leads to high blood glucose levels. This might cause insulin resistance in body cells and, in worst case scenarios, it might trigger the immune system to attack the pancreas. High insulin levels in the blood might trigger memory loss and might even induce a coma.

Diabetes. Amylin deficiency leads to the overproduction of insulin, which, in the long run, impairs the pancreas. When the normal working of the pancreas is damaged, diabetes may develop.

Weight gain. Amylin deficiency promotes insulin resistance. When body cells become insensitive to insulin, there is less sugar converted into energy. So, the blood glucose level remains high. Insulin is responsible for carrying off these sugars to be stored as fats. Instead of these sugars being used as energy, they end up being stored as fat in the cells, which is the start of weight gain.

Headache. Thanks to insulin resistance, the body cells lack a reliable source of energy, which causes the body to switch to burning fats as an alternative energy source. One of the side effects of this process is normally headache and nausea.

The Insulin Resistance Diet

Insulin resistance causes slower absorption of sugars into body cells. This condition is rampant in obese people and diabetics. It is projected that the number of diabetics in the next 20 years will be over 320 million. This indicates a very worrying trend of diabetes. One of the things we can do to fight against diabetes is to improve our diet. Studies have shown that weight loss is a very effective means of minimizing insulin resistance. Here are the components of an insulin resistant diet:

Low carbs. Food high in carbs are responsible for blood sugar spikes. High levels of blood glucose promote insulin resistance. To ensure a stable blood glucose level, you should stick to low-carb foods.

Avoid sugary drinks. The American Diabetes Association advises against consumption of sugary drinks. These drinks with high sugar content include fruit juice, corn syrup, and other concentrates. Sugary drinks have a high sugar content, and they spike blood sugar levels. So, it'd be prudent to stay away from sugary drinks.

More fiber. Fiber is important in reducing the blood glucose levels. It improves the digestive health and improves blood circulation.

Healthy fats. Monounsaturated fats are very critical in improving heart health and regulating insulin levels.

Protein. Studies show that dietary protein is beneficial for people who suffer from diabetes. Regular consumption of protein is important for muscle growth and bone mass.

Size. Instead of taking large servings of a meal, opt for smaller portions of food, so that your post-meal blood glucose levels may be stable.

The Best Food for Diabetics

Diabetics don't have the luxury of eating any food they might want. For instance, sugar-laden foods and high-fat foods would spike their blood sugar levels and worsen the condition. They should instead stick to foods that are sources of minerals and vitamins. Foods like:

Fish. Fish is an important source of omega-3 fatty acids. These fatty acids are especially great for people with heart health complications and those who are at risk of stroke. Omega three fatty acids also protect your blood vessels, as well as reduce inflammation. Studies show that people who consume fish on the regular have better heart health than those who don't.

Greens. They are very nutritious and have low calories. Leafy greens like kale and spinach are excellent sources of minerals and vitamins. Leafy greens reduce inflammation markers, as well improve blood pressure. They are also high in antioxidants.

Eggs. The good old egg has been abused at the hands of intellectual conmen who have long said, albeit incorrectly, that eggs are bad. Eggs are excellent for reducing heart disease complications and also decreasing inflammation markers. Regular consumption of eggs improves cholesterol and blood glucose levels.

Chia seeds. They are high in fiber, and this fiber is critical in lowering blood glucose levels as well as in slowing down the rate of movement of food along the gut.

Nuts. Nuts are both tasty and healthy. They are great sources of fiber and are low in carbs. Regular consumption improves heart health and reduces inflammation and improves blood circulation.

Summary

Type 2 diabetes is a degenerative disease that impairs the ability of the pancreas to produce insulin. The hormone insulin is produced by the pancreas, and its main function is to regulate the conversion of glucose to energy. The risk of developing diabetes can be greatly minimized by taking the two steps: losing weight and having a balanced diet. The number of people with diabetes is at an all-time high, and people in both developed and poor countries are battling the disease. Symptoms of type 2 diabetes include tiredness, never-ending thirst, the constant urge to pee, irritability, weak immune system, and shivering. A carbohydrate metabolism test determines how blood sugar reacts to fasting. During a fast, blood sugar levels go up. Supplements are necessary for supplying important nutrients that may not be in the diet. The intake of supplements should be daily for optimum results. The important supplements include sodium, potassium, magnesium, zinc, calcium, and iodine. These are some of the measures to take to keep insulin levels low: have a strict diet, consume small portions, exercise regularly, and drink water constantly.

Chapter 12: Fasting For Heart Health

How Fasting Improves Your Heart's Health

Numerous studies have shown that fasting has a positive impact on heart health. Many people who have gone on a fast have reported feeling energetic and livelier afterward, which could be attributed to improved blood flow and general heart health. However, you need to fast consistently to achieve results.

Improves your heartbeat. When you go on a fast, your body is free from the digestion load, and so it channels that energy into optimizing your physiological functions. Your heart stands to gain from the optimized body functions, especially improving your heartbeat.

Improves blood pressure. Studies show that fasting has a positive impact on blood pressure. The rate of blood pressure is affected by factors like weight gain and obesity. But since fasting helps in weight loss, it has the extended advantage of lowering blood pressure, which improves the overall heart health.

Reduces cholesterol. Regularly fasting helps in lowering bad cholesterol. Also, controlled fasting increases the base metabolic rate.

Improved blood vessel health. Fasting is critical in improving the health of blood vessels. When blood vessels are subjected to high blood pressure, they slowly start to wear out, and might eventually burst up—which could be fatal, especially in the case of arteries. But fasting helps reduce blood pressure and bad cholesterol. The result is improved blood flow and overall heart health.

Autophagy. Regular dry fasts trigger the body to digest its weak and damaged cells in a process known as autophagy. Cell autophagy is very crucial because it helps eliminate old and damaged cells and creates room for new cells. With a new batch of cells to work with, the heart health is given a tremendous boost.

Summary

Fasting has been shown to improve the health of the heart. When you are fasting, your body reserves energy that would have gone into digestion for purposes of improving the heart health. It can execute its physiological functions much better. Fasting has also been shown to improve blood pressure. Fasting helps reduce obesity and reduces weight gain. This causes massive improvement in blood pressure. Fasting also plays a critical role in reducing cholesterol. Bad cholesterol increases the rate of developing heart disease. Also, controlled fasting increases the base metabolic rate. Fasting also improves the health of blood vessels. High blood pressure might cause blood vessels to wear out slowly, but fasting has a restorative effect on the blood vessels. Fasting also allows the body to digest its weak cells and make room for new and powerful body cells.

Chapter 13: The General Results of Fasting

Positive Effects of Fasting

You will get varied results depending on your preferred method of fasting, whether it's intermittent fasting, alternate-day, or prolonged fasting. These are some of the positive effects of fasting:

Weight loss. Fasting is an efficient way of losing weight. A study in 2015 showed that alternate fasting for a week resulted in weight loss of up to seven percent. When your body uses up the glucose in your blood, it now turns to the fat reserves to power its bodily functions. This helps in achieving weight loss.

Release of the human growth hormone. The human growth hormone promotes the growth of muscles and reduces obesity. Fasting triggers the secretion of the human growth hormone. This hormone is very crucial in building your body cells.

Improves insulin sensitivity. Low insulin sensitivity restricts the absorption of sugars into body cells. This might lead to complications such as chronic weight gain. Fasting leads to high insulin sensitivity that helps in absorption of sugars into body cells.

Normalizes ghrelin levels. Ghrelin is the hunger hormone which sends out hunger signals. Most obese people have abnormal ghrelin hormone levels that keep them in a perpetual state of hunger. Fasting, however, remedies this situation by normalizing ghrelin hormone levels, and thus you can receive accurate signals about hunger.

Lowers triglyceride levels. Depriving yourself of food for a set period of time has the effect of lowering bad cholesterol, and in the process, triglycerides are reduced.

Slows down aging. Many studies have shown the link between fasting and increased longevity in animals. Fasting allows the body to cleanse itself, promotes cell autophagy, and in the long run, lengthens lifespan.

Negative Effects of Fasting

As much as fasting is a practice with many benefits, admittedly there is a dark side too. These are some of the negative effects of fasting:

Strained body. A prolonged fast might put a big deal of a strain on your body. This may alter—albeit slightly—the normal processes of your body. A prolonged fast might slow down the effectiveness of your body as the body adapts to survive on too little energy.

Headaches. Headaches are common during fasts, especially at the start. The headache is normally a response of the brain to diminished blood glucose levels that force the body to switch to burning fats as a source of energy.

Low blood pressure. Fasting is a major cause of low blood pressure. Low blood pressure slows down the conversion of sugars into energy. This may lead to complications such as temporary blindness and, in extreme cases, can induce a coma.

Eating disorders. For someone who's too eager, it is easy to abuse fasting and turn it into an eating disorder. The main aim of fasting is to improve health, but starving yourself and having an eating disorder is anything but healthy. Some of the eating disorders that people who fast are at risk of developing include anorexia and bulimia.

Cravings. The hunger triggered by fasting might cause us to overcompensate. We may develop cravings for fast foods and other unhealthy foods. During our eating window, we may find ourselves consuming a lot of unhealthy foods, under the delusion that the fast will override that.

Summary

Weight loss is one of the main benefits of fasting. When you fast, your blood glucose is diminished, and this forces your body to turn to fats as an alternative source of energy. Fasting also promotes the production of the human growth hormone. This is the hormone responsible for muscle growth. Fasting also improves insulin sensitivity. Low insulin sensitivity impairs the body's ability to convert sugars into energy. Fasting also leads to high insulin sensitivity that helps in the absorption of sugars into body cells. Fasting also helps normalize ghrelin levels. The ghrelin hormone is known as the hunger hormone. Most obese people have abnormally high ghrelin levels that give incorrect hunger signals and make the obese person perpetually hungry. Fasting helps in correcting this problem, and the obese person starts to receive accurate signals. The negative effects of fasting include straining the body, headaches, low blood pressure, and eating disorders.

PART 4.4

Important Factors that Improve the Quality of Fasting

Chapter 14: Nutrition

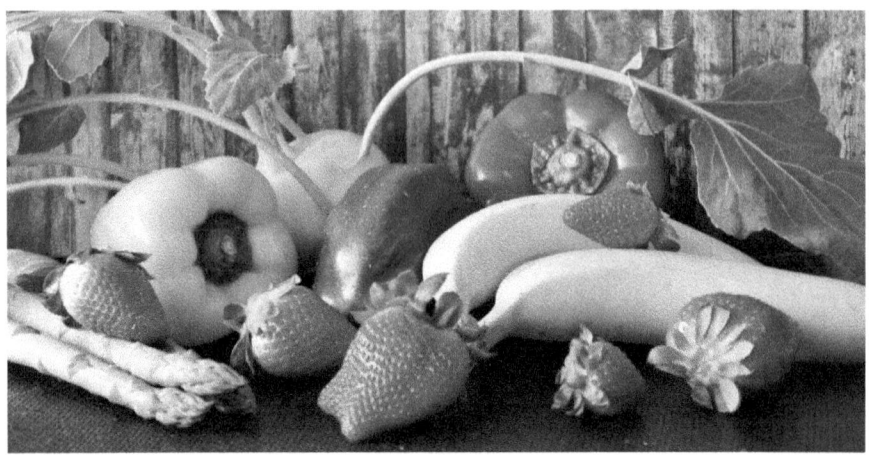

What Constitutes Good Nutrition?

Good nutrition implies a diet that contains all the required and important nutrients in appropriate proportions. When you fail to observe good nutrition, you risk developing complications from certain nutrient deficiencies. A good nutrition shouldn't be a one-off thing, but it should be a part of your lifestyle.

A great nutrition minimizes the risk of developing health complications such as diabetes, heart disease, and chronic weight gain. Here are the most important constituents of great nutrition:

- **Protein**

This nutrient is very important for muscle health, skin health, and hair. Also, it assists in the bodily reactions. Amino acids are essential for human growth and protein is stacked with amino acids. The best sources of protein include fish, eggs, and lentils.

- **Carbohydrates**

Carbohydrates are the main sources of energy for the body. They provide sugars that are converted into energy. There are two classes of carbohydrates: simple and complex. Simple carbohydrates are digested easily, and complex carbohydrates take time. Fruits and grains are some of the main sources of simple carbohydrates whereas beans and vegetables are sources of complex carbohydrates. For proper digestion, dietary fiber (carbohydrate) is needed. Men need a daily intake of 30 grams of fiber and women need 24 grams. Important sources of dietary fiber include legumes and whole grains.

- **Fats**

Fats play an essential role in health improvement. Both monounsaturated and polyunsaturated fats are healthy. Sources of monounsaturated fats include avocados and nuts. As for polyunsaturated fats, seafood is a major source. Unhealthy fats include trans fats and saturated fats, mostly found in junk food.

- **Vitamins**

Vitamins A, B, C, D, E, and K are necessary for the body's optimal functioning. A deficiency in the important vitamins can lead to serious health complications and weakened immune system.

- **Minerals**

Calcium, iron, zinc, and iodine are some of the essential minerals. They are found in a variety of foods including vegetables, grains, and meats.

- **Water**

Most of the human body is composed of water. It is a very essential nutrient for the proper functioning of the body.

Why Good Nutrition Is Important

The main reason why people ensure that they have a good nutrition is to improve their health. A good nutrition is essentially about consuming foods that are rich in vitamins, minerals, and fats. So, here are some of the reasons why good nutrition is vital.

Reduces risk of cancer. Good nutrition plays a vital role in optimizing your health. If you consume healthy food, you drastically reduce your chances of getting cancer, as many cancers are a result of bad lifestyle choices.

Reduces risk of developing high blood pressure. High blood pressure causes a strain on the heart. It also leads to the wearing and tearing of the blood vessels. Having good nutrition normalizes your blood pressure and thus improves your heart health.

Lowers cholesterol. Bad cholesterol leads to serious complications like heart disease. When you observe good nutrition that involves fruits and essential vitamins, the bad cholesterol is eliminated, thus improving the functioning of your body.

Increased energy. Bad food choices have a draining effect. However, nutritious foods replenish the body cells with vital nutrients, and thus the body is active. A nutritious diet is a key to improving productivity.

Improved immunity. Diseases are always looking for new victims. People who have a poor diet are bound to have a weak immune system. The weak immune system won't sufficiently protect them against attacks. On the other hand, people who consume a nutritious diet tend to have a strong immune system. This improved immunity keeps diseases at bay.

The Advantages of a High-Fat Diet

Many studies have shown that a low-carb, high-fat diet has many health benefits, including weight management, and reduced risk of diabetes, cancer, and Alzheimer's. A high-fat diet is characterized by low carbohydrate intake and high intake of fat. The low carbohydrate intake puts the body into ketosis, a condition that optimizes burning of fat and helps convert fat into ketone bodies that act as an energy source of the brain. These are some of the advantages of a high-fat diet:

Stronger immune system. Saturated fats are an ally of the immune system. They help fight off microbes, viruses, and fungi. Fats help in the fight against diseases. A great source of saturated fats includes butter and coconut.

Improves skin health and eyesight. When someone is lacking in fatty acids, they are likely to develop dry skin and eyes. Fatty acids help in improving skin elasticity and strengthening eyesight.

Lowers risk of heart disease. Saturated fats trigger production of good cholesterol, which is key in reducing the risk of heart disease. Saturated fats also help fight inflammation. A good source of saturated fats includes eggs and coconut oil.

Strong bones. Healthy fats improve the density of bones and thus minimize the risk of bone diseases. Fats promote healthy calcium metabolism. Fatty acids, too, play a critical role in minimizing the risk of bone complications such as osteoporosis.

Improves reproductive health. Fats play a critical role in the production of hormones that improve fertility in both men and women. A high-fat diet improves reproductive health and, in particular, the production of testosterone and estrogen.

Weight loss. A high-fat diet promotes high metabolism and, as a result, the body can crunch more calories, leading to weight loss.

Improved muscle gain. A high-fat diet promotes muscle gain. This is achieved through hormone production and speeding up cell recovery after strenuous exercise.

Role of Ketone Bodies

The three ketone bodies produced by the liver include acetoacetate, beta-hydroxybutyrate, and acetone. Ketone bodies are water-soluble, and it takes a blood or urine test to determine their levels.

Ketone bodies are oxidized in the mitochondria to provide energy. The heart uses fatty acids as fuel in normal circumstances, but during ketogenesis, it switches to ketone bodies. When the blood glucose levels are high, the body stores the excesses as fat. When you go for an extended period of time without eating, the blood glucose levels diminish. This triggers the body to convert fat into usable energy. Most body cells can utilize fatty acids, except the brain. The liver thus converts fats into ketone bodies and releases them into the blood to supply energy to the brain. When ketone bodies start to build up in the blood, problems might arise. An increase in the levels of acetone can induce acidosis, a condition where blood pH is lowered. Acidosis has a negative impact on most of the body cells, and in worst cases, it leads to death. With that in mind, it is prudent to replenish your body with carbohydrates as soon as ketosis kicks off. A person with type 1 diabetes is more susceptible to high levels of ketone bodies. For instance, when they fail to take an insulin shot, they will experience hypoglycemia. The combination of low blood glucose level and high glucagon level will cause the liver to produce ketone bodies at an alarming rate which might cause complications.

Benefits of the Ketogenic Diet

Here are some of the benefits associated with ketone bodies:

Treating Alzheimer's. Alzheimer's behaves in a way similar to diabetes. Essentially, it is the brain resisting insulin. Due to insulin resistance, the brain only gets minimal energy, which might cause the death of brain cells. However, ketone bodies are an alternative source of energy that the brain can utilize. Ketone bodies have been shown to prevent a buildup of compounds that enhance the development of Alzheimer.

Normalizes insulin production. Ketone bodies are only produced when blood glucose is low. For this reason, the pancreas stops pumping more insulin to aid in the absorption of sugars because the body has already switched into ketogenesis.

Regulates metabolism. Ketone bodies regulate metabolism through their effects on mitochondria. The mitochondria are the cells' power plants, and they respond better to energy from fats rather than glucose. In this sense, ketone bodies improve the functioning of the mitochondria.

Lowers hunger. When the body is utilizing ketone bodies, it seems that there's less of an urge to consume food. Ketogenesis regulates the hunger hormone. When a person is consuming fast foods, there is no end to the urge to take another serving. Eventually, this leads to weight gain.

Increases good cholesterol. The good cholesterol improves blood flow and the condition of your heart. Ketogenesis helps in the production of the good cholesterol and thus helps in improving heart health.

Improves brain health. Ketone bodies are especially effective as a source of energy for the brain. Many people who have practiced the ketone diet say that it improves their mental clarity and focus.

The Importance of a Well-Balanced Diet

When we talk about a balanced diet, we refer to a variety of foods that supply us with important nutrients such as protein, carbohydrates, healthy fats, vitamins, and minerals. So, what is the importance of a well-balanced diet?

Strengthens immune system. When you consume a diet that's rich in nutrients, your immune system will become stronger. This places your body in a far better place to fight disease vectors that might have otherwise overwhelmed your body's defense system.

Weight loss. In the past, obesity was a problem in only developed nations. Not anymore. Nowadays even poor people are struggling with obesity. This is partially due to fast foods being cheaper and more convenient. As you can imagine, obesity has become a crisis the world over. The open secret is that obesity can be mitigated through a balanced diet. A diet rich in nutritious elements will nourish your body and also regulate your appetite so that you don't fall into the temptation of eating unhealthy foods.

Mental health. People who observe a balanced diet are less likely to fall into bad moods and depression. The nutritious elements stabilize their emotions and enable them to be more resistant to the autosuggestions of their mind.

Skin health. Dry skin is often the result of a bad diet. When you have a balanced diet, your skin and hair are nourished, and it gives you a glow. Foods rich in vitamins and collagen improve skin elasticity.

Promotes growth. A balanced diet helps kids have a well-formed body as they transition into adults and it helps adults maintain a well-figured body.

Summary

A good nutrition is a diet that contains all the important nutrients in appropriate portions. You risk developing complications if you fail to follow a good nutrition. The risk of developing health complications is greatly minimized by a great nutrition. Protein is one of the most important elements of a good nutrition. It is important for muscle health, skin health and development of hair. Protein also plays a role in bodily reactions. Carbohydrates are the major source of energy. They provide glucose that the body cells use to power activities of the body. Fats also play an important role in improving health. Monounsaturated fats and polyunsaturated fats are especially healthy. Vitamins are necessary for the body to function optimally. Minerals and water are important too. People ensure that they have good nutrition to improve their health. They achieve this by consuming foods that are rich in nutritious elements. A high-fat diet promotes strong immunity, better eyesight, a lower risk of heart disease, and stronger bones.

Chapter 15: Exercise

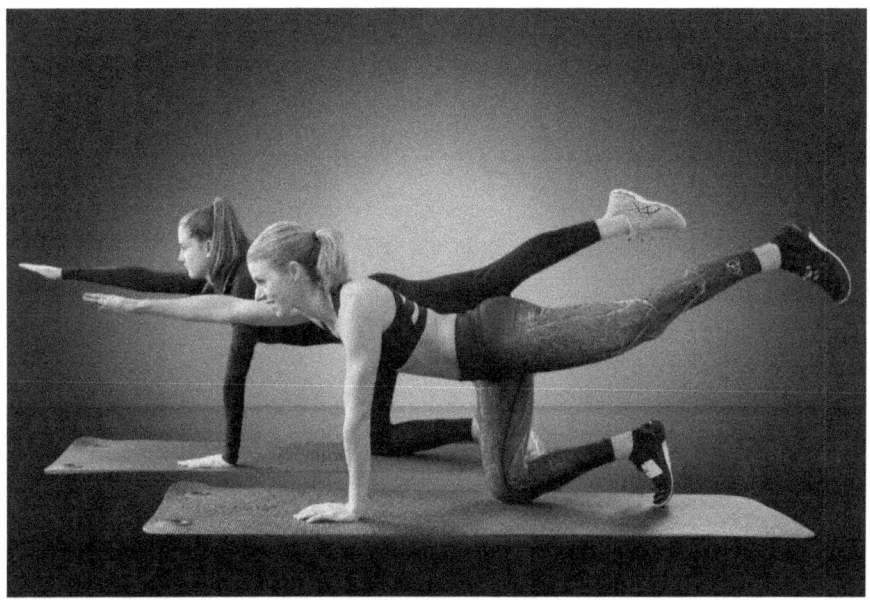

Pros of Exercising While Fasting

For the longest time, it was considered unhealthy to exercise while on a fast, but new evidence has shown that it is perfectly healthy to exercise even while you are fasting.

When you fast for health purposes, it shows that you are committed to improving your health and managing your weight. One of the ways you could get better results is by turning to physical exercise. A combination of intermittent fasting and physical exercise will burn up calories and help you reach your health goals in the shortest time possible.

The time of day that you exercise seems to affect the outcome. For instance, exercising in the morning right after you wake up promotes more weight loss than exercising at night. For intermittent fasting to be effective, you need to abstain from food for at least 16 hours.

When you exercise while on a fast, you speed up weight loss and optimize your health because of increased oxidation that promotes the growth of muscle cells.

It enriches your blood. Exercising has a positive effect on your breathing system and lung capacity. This helps in increasing the oxygen levels in your blood.

Exercising also improves heart health. Aerobic exercises, in particular, improve blood circulation and develop the stamina of the heart. Now, the blood pressure stabilizes and nutrients can spread to the whole body.

Exercising while on a fast improves your body's adaptability. It is never a good idea to idle around while on a fast, as it will trigger cravings. However, when you engage in physical activity, your body starts to adapt. It helps you create more stamina to endure your fast.

Best Exercises to Do

Exercising while fasting increases the rate of calorie burning. As a result, more weight is lost, and health is optimized in much less time. Here are the best exercises to perform while on a fast:

- **Aerobic exercise**

Aerobic exercise increases your heartbeat and breathing cycle. Aerobic exercise also improves lung capacity and heart health. Some of the benefits of aerobic exercise include improved mental health, minimized inflammation, lowered blood pressure, lowered blood sugar, and a minimized risk of heart disease, stroke, type 2 diabetes, and cancer. Aerobic exercises tend to be intense and easy to perform. Some examples of aerobic exercises include dancing, speed-walking, jogging, and cycling.

- **Strength training**

Strength training is important for muscle gain. People who perform strength training have more energy and keep their bodies at peak performance. Strength training improves your mental health, decreases blood sugar levels, enhances weight management, corrects posture, increases balance, and relieves pain in the back and joints. Strength training may be performed either in the gym or at home. Professional guidance depends on the exact exercise and equipment required. Strength training mostly takes the form of exercises such as pull-ups, push-ups, sit-ups, squats, and lunges. It is recommended to take breaks from strength training to allow muscle growth.

- **Stretching**

Stretching exercises are vital in improving the flexibility of a person. The exercises are designed to improve the strength and flexibility of tendons. Stretching exercises also improve the aesthetic quality of muscles. They also improve the circulation of blood and promote nourishment of all body cells.

- **Balance exercises**

Balance exercises promote agility. The exercises are designed to make your joints flexible. Balance exercises lead to improved focus and motor skills. The exercises include squats, sit-ups, and leg lifts.

Summary

Contrary to what people thought for the longest time, it is healthy to exercise while on a fast. A combination of exercise and fasting is a resource-intensive activity that makes your body burn more calories. Studies show that exercising in the morning has a far better outcome than exercising at night before bed. When you exercise while fasting, oxidation in cells promotes the growth of muscles. Exercising while on a fast also enriches your blood. The improved breathing cycle and lung capacity help in increasing the level of oxygen in the blood. Exercising is vital in improving heart health and blood circulation. It is never a good idea to stay idle while you are on a fast. Your hunger will be magnified, and it might cause to break the fast. Some of the best exercises to do for maximum weight loss and health improvement include aerobic exercises, strength training, stretching and balance exercises.

Chapter 16: Having a Partner to Keep You in Check

Role of a Partner

Depriving yourself of food is by no means easy. If you have no experience, the temptation to slide back is real. In some instances, fasting might make you lapse into a worse state than before. This is especially after a small duration of fasting where the hunger is extreme, and then you are tempted into eating unhealthy foods, trapping you into eating them.

Having a partner to keep you in check is a good step, and if they are into fasting themselves, that's even better. Ideally, your partner should be someone that "understands" you. He or she will make fasting less taxing. They will be there to see your progress and offer constructive criticism when needed. As your fasting progresses, they will help you adjust accordingly or make tweaks, to go through the fast in the safest manner possible.

Your partner will hold you accountable for your fasting journey. Attaining health goals is no easy task. It takes dedication, discipline, and consistency. It's exactly why you need a partner to hold you accountable when you stray or when you fall back on your goals. A responsible partner will be interested in your gains (i.e., asking questions about your weight loss so far and wanting to know what your diet is like).

A partner is also important because you have someone to talk to about your journey. They can offer you psychosocial support in your moments of vulnerability. It makes a world of difference. And you will stick to your goals knowing that someone cares.

Traits to Look for in a Partner

Not everyone may qualify to be a partner to someone who's fasting. The first thing to look out for is their opinion on the subject of fasting. Some people seem to think that fasting is a bad practice and a waste of time. Clearly, you wouldn't want such a person as your partner.

- **Patience**

Your partner should demonstrate patience. You cannot rush things while fasting. Sometimes, the results might take time, and in such situations, the last thing you want is someone on your neck, probably trashing your methods.

- **Observation skills**

A great partner must be a good observer. Their job is to spot loopholes that need to be closed, to assess situations, and to weigh overall progress. They need strong observation skills that will make them suitable for their positions. Also, remember that it is sometimes critical to call off a fast. Maybe you will be hard on yourself even when you are falling apart. An observant partner should notice the change and suggest that you stop.

- **Communication skills**

They should have good communication skills. What good is it to know something and not express it in a timely and appropriate fashion? A great partner should be very communicative and should express him/herself in an elaborate manner.

- **Knowledgeable**

A good partner should be knowledgeable. They should have a working knowledge of the whole subject of fasting. During every step of the fast, they should have a mental picture of what's coming. This will strengthen your bond and together you can meet any challenge.

- **Respect**

They should be able to respect you, your methods, and also have self-respect. This creates an enabling environment.

Should You Join A Support Group?

When your brain floods you with hunger hormones during a fast, the temptation to quit is real. One of the methods to minimize your chances of quitting is to join a support group. This is ideally a group of people who have similar fasting pursuits as you. Now you have a family to keep you in check and boost your confidence.

A support network will allow you to cope and express your feelings and get connected with like-minded people. In times of vulnerability, others will come to your help. As other members share their experiences, you learn that you are not alone, and you even broaden your perspective and wisdom.

Support networks include people who are at various stages toward the common goal you all have. In times of conflict, you have ready help, and if you are at an advanced stage yourself, then you should offer help to those in need of it too. Support networks have non-judgmental environments and therapeutic effects.

The best support groups are those that foster frequent get-togethers. Ideally, the members should come from the same society, but that doesn't mean other kinds of support groups are necessary. For instance, you could join an online support network and be free to commune with your family at your convenience. Online support groups seem to be a thing nowadays. People from around the world with common goals are coming together to form support networks.

The most important thing when you join a support group is to become a giver rather than a taker. Or both. When everyone is interested in giving, you have a resourceful group of like-minded people.

Summary

People who are overwhelmed by the idea of staying without food should consider getting a partner. Your partner should help you cultivate a strong sense of discipline and stick to your routine. Ideally, your partner should be someone who understands you. He or she will help you get through fasting. A supportive partner is there to check your progress and offer constructive criticism when the occasion calls for it. He or she should be someone that you can open up to and express your fears and concerns. With the right partner, your fasting journey will be smooth and enjoyable.

Your partner should be patient, observant, communicative, respectful, and knowledgeable. Joining a support group will help you come together with other like-minded people for a common goal. You are guaranteed of ready help and psychosocial support. The best support group to join should comprise of people from your local area, but it doesn't rule out joining even online support groups and communing with people from different parts of the world.

Chapter 17: Motivation

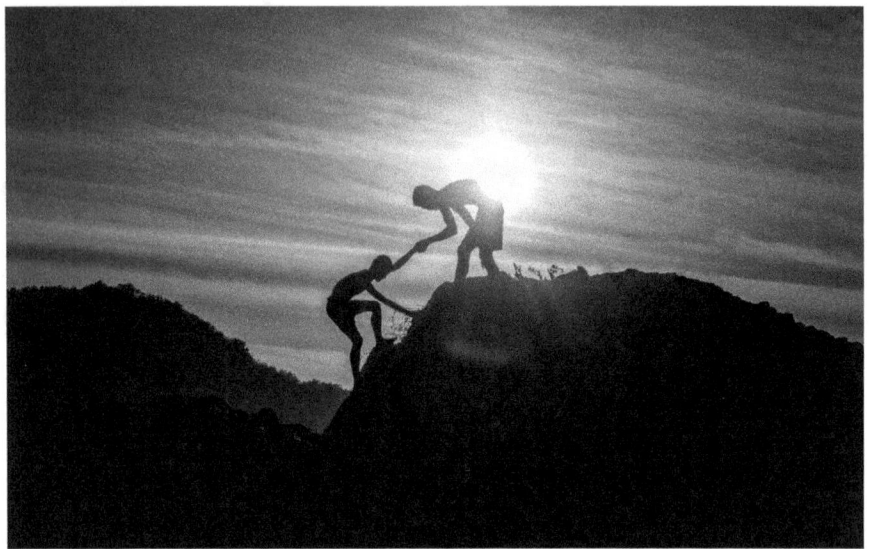

How to Stay Motivated Throughout Your Fast

Get a partner. If you go it alone, you are much more likely to forgive yourself and tweak the fast to suit you. For that reason, let there be a person to whom you are accountable. This person should put you in check and ensure that you follow the rules. Offer constructive criticism, and suggestions. A partner will help you stick to your routine. The ideal partner should be patient, empathetic, a good communicator, and knowledgeable about fasting. Let them share in your accomplishments as much as they have shared in your trials and struggle.

Seek knowledge. Being informed makes all the difference. You will know every possible outcome. You are aware of all the side effects of fasting and how to persist through the unpleasant experience instead of just quitting. Knowledge will help you optimize your fast and make you reap more benefits than anyone who had just deprived themselves of food. Being knowledgeable is important also in the sense that you are more aware of when to stop.

Set goals. Don't get into fasting with mental blindness. Instead, make an effort to set milestones. When you achieve a goal—for instance, when you hit your target weight—celebrate and then go back to reducing weight. Your brain responds to victory by making you feel confident. Now, you will have more confidence in your capacity to withstand hunger.

Develop positivity. A positive attitude makes all the difference. Keep reading about successful people who have achieved what you are looking for. Lockout all the negative energies that would derail you.

Record your progress. It is easy to underestimate yourself. As long as you keep going, the achievements will always be there. It's just a matter of recognizing them and celebrating.

How to Make Fasting Your Lifestyle

There are different approaches to fasting. You may fast every other day, once a week, or even a couple of times every month. In each instance, there are benefits.

But if you'd like to reap great benefits out of fasting, you should purposefully make it a daily ritual. Many people in the world today fast on a daily basis and have reported an increased quality of life.

The most common and most rewarding method is the 16:8 intermittent fasting. In this method, you fast for 16 hours in a day and then eat during the other 8 hours to complete the cycle.

Ideally, when you wake up, you should take a drink of water or black coffee and either exercise or just go on about your work. At around noon, your eating window opens, and you're free to have your meals up until 8 pm when the eating window closes.

During this eight-hour eating window, it is common to be tempted to overeat or indulge in unhealthy foods, thinking that the coming fast will "take care of that." Well, you must be careful not to fall into this temptation, or else your gains will be negated. Consume healthy and nutritious foods during the eating window and adhere to your 16-hour fast. The weight loss starts occurring in as short a span as a few days.

If you incorporate intermittent fasting into your lifestyle, the weight loss keeps going until you hit a stable weight where it plateaus. When fasting is your lifestyle, it makes your health improvement and weight loss permanent.

Summary

You need to take a few measures to stay motivated throughout the fast. One of the measures is to get a partner. A partner should hold you accountable and keep you in check so that you don't stray from the fasting routine. The ideal partner should be patient, empathetic, and a good communicator. Another way of motivating yourself is through seeking knowledge. As a knowledgeable person, you will be aware of all the responses that your body will give off. Knowledge will also help you optimize your fast and get the best possible results. Other ways to stay motivated throughout the fast include setting goals, developing positivity and recording your progress. If you make fasting part of your lifestyle, you stand to reap more benefits. The most common and most efficient fasting method is the 16:8, where you fast for 16 hours and then have an eating window of 8 hours.

Chapter 18: Foods for the Fast

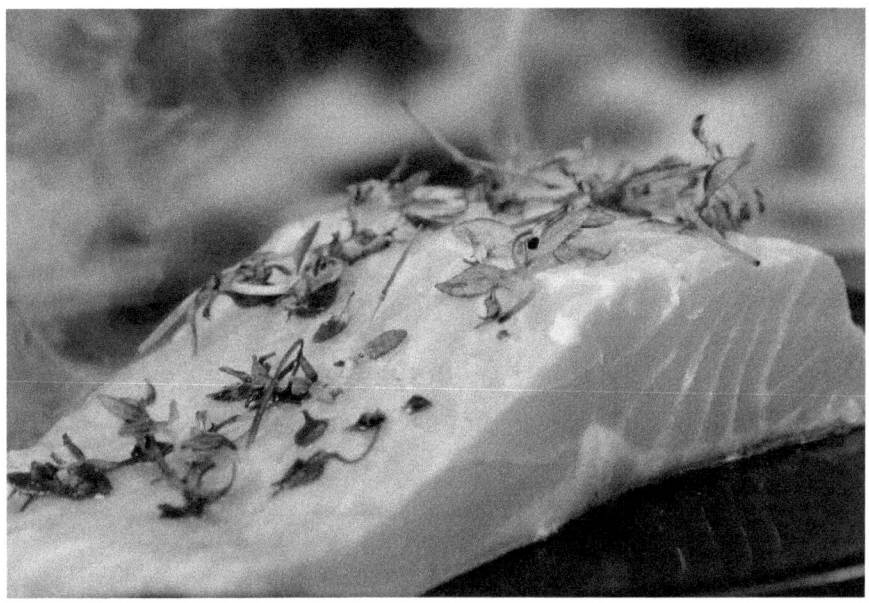

How Food Controls the Rate of the Success of Fasting

Depriving yourself of food is no easy task. Your body will tune up the hunger, and you will have to suppress the urge to feed. Not easy.

When you consume food, it is digested and released into the bloodstream as sugars. The pancreas secretes the hormone insulin to help in absorption of these sugars into body cells. When you stay for long without eating, there is no more food getting digested, and thus no more sugars getting released into the blood. The body soon runs out of the existing sugars and meets a crisis. The body is forced to switch to fats to provide energy for various physiological functions.

The foods that you eat have a massive impact on the efficacy of the fast. If you take light meals or small portions of food during the eating window, you will experience a higher degree of hunger during the fast. On the other side, if you consume large amounts of food during your eating window, your hunger will not be as intense.

One of the tricks to reducing hunger during the fast is to consume foods that are high in dietary fiber. Such foods make you full for a long time and will thus minimize the unpleasant feeling triggered by hunger.

Consuming healthy foods during your eating window is important. Some people fall into the temptation of eating unhealthy foods or even eating too much, and the effect is negative.

Intermittent fasting is favored by many people because it doesn't restrict consumption of foods, unlike fad diets that insist on vegan meals or raw food.

The Worst Foods to Take During Fasting

If you want to speed up your weight loss and avoid lifestyle diseases, these are some of the foods to cut back on, or maybe stay away from:

Sugary drinks. The high dose of fructose in sugary drinks will cause an extreme surge of blood sugar levels. High amounts of this kind of sugar promote insulin resistance and liver disease. High levels of insulin resistance have a negative impact on the absorption of sugars into body cells. This creates the perfect recipe for the development of heart disease and diabetes.

Junk food. They might taste heavenly, but the ingredients of most junk foods come from hell. Junk foods have almost zero nutritional value. Fries are prepared using hydrogenated oil that contains trans fats. Studies have been made on trans fats, and the conclusion is that continued consumption of trans fats leads to heart complications and cancer.

Processed food. Most processed foods have a long shelf life thanks to a host of nasty chemicals poured into them. The processed foods are made durable to gain a commercial edge over organic products with a limited shelf life. Most processed foods are high in sugars, sodium, and have low fiber content and nutrients.

White bread and cakes. Baked goods tend to affect people with celiac disease, most especially. But more than that, most of these baked goods are stashed with processed ingredients—sugars and fats—and they are low on fiber. Most baked goods trigger abnormal surges in blood sugar levels and increase the risk of heart disease.

Alcohol. Studies show that alcohol induces inflammation on the liver. Excessive alcohol consumption will eliminate all the successes of your fast and promote weight gain and even development of diabetes.

Seed oils. Studies show that these oils are unnatural. They contain harmful fatty acids that increase the risk of developing heart complications.

The Best Foods to Take During Fasting

These are some of the best foods to indulge in while you fast to reach your important health goals:

Nuts. Nuts are rich in nutritional value. Almonds, Brazil nuts, lentils, oatmeal, etc. have properties that help in the production of good cholesterol. Good cholesterol promotes heart health. Nuts are excellent sources of vitamins and minerals. Oatmeal, in particular, is essential in normalizing blood glucose levels.

Fruits and greens. They are important sources of essential nutrients that improve both gut health and brain health. Broccoli is rich in phytonutrients that reduce the risk of heart complications and cancers. Apples contain antioxidants that eliminate harmful radicals. Kale contains the vital vitamin K. Blueberries are excellent sources of fiber and phytonutrients. Avocados are good sources of monounsaturated fats that lower bad cholesterol and improve heart health.

White meats. These are an excellent source of protein and fatty acids. Fish provide omega-3 fatty acids which improve heart health and stimulate muscle growth. Chicken is a great source of protein, and it promotes the growth of muscle cells.

Grains. They are excellent sources of protein and dietary fiber that will keep you full. Grains also help in improving heart health and normalizing blood pressure.

Eggs. Eggs are excellent sources of protein, and they tend to fill you up thus minimizing hunger levels.

Tubers. Foods such as potatoes and sweet potatoes are loaded with essential vitamins and carbohydrates.

Dairy. Dairy seems to reduce the risk of development of obesity and type 2 diabetes. Cheese and whole milk are excellent sources of protein and essential minerals that promote bone development.

Summary

When you go on a fast, your body increases the hunger levels in an attempt to pressure you to look for food. Staying without food for a long time causes the body to switch to fats as an alternative energy source. When the carbohydrates supplying energy to the brain are depleted, the liver produces ketone bodies to supply energy to the brain. The food you eat (and the portion) will impact your hunger levels during the fast. It is important to consume healthy foods during the eating window no matter how strong the temptation to stray is. Some of the worst foods that you can indulge in while fasting includes sugary drinks, junk foods, processed foods, white bread and cakes, alcohol, and seed oils. On the other hand, some of the best foods you can indulge in would be nuts, fruits and greens, white meat, grains, eggs, tubes, and dairy.

Conclusion

Thanks for making it through to the end of *Strength Training*, let's hope it was informative and able to provide you with all of the tools you need to achieve your goals whatever it is that they may be. Just because you've finished this book doesn't mean there is nothing left to learn on the topic. Expanding your horizons is the only way to find the mastery you seek.

The next step is to stop reading and to get started doing whatever it is that you need to do to ensure that you will be able to get stronger and leaner. If you find that you still need help getting started, you will likely have better results by creating a schedule that you hope to follow, including strict deadlines for various parts of the tasks as well as the overall completion of your preparations such as writing down your strength goals and how your ideal body looks like. It is an important passage that works like magic if done correctly.

Studies show that when training is broken down into individual pieces, including individual deadlines, people have a much greater chance of sticking to it and achieving goals compared to someone that has a general need of being fit but no real timetable for doing so. Even if it seems silly, go ahead and set your own deadlines for reaching your goals, complete with indicators of success and failure. After you have successfully completed all of your required preparations, you will be glad that you did.

Once you have finished your initial preparations, it is important to understand that they are just that: only part of a larger plan of preparation. Your best chances for overall success will come by taking the time to learn as many ways to train your strength as possible. Only by using your prepared status as a springboard to greater preparation will you be able to truly rest soundly knowing that you are prepared for anything and everything that life decides to throw at you. Because, at the end of the day, remember that training in the gym is not only a way to get a better body, but also to become the strongest version of yourself.

www.ingramcontent.com/pod-product-compliance
Lightning Source LLC
LaVergne TN
LVHW010331070526
838199LV00065B/5725